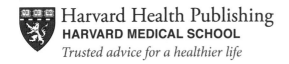

Harvard Health Publishing
HARVARD MEDICAL SCHOOL
Trusted advice for a healthier life

Dear Reader,

How many times have you used your shoulders today? Think about it. Every time you reach for a cup on a high shelf, wave to a friend, raise your coffee mug to take a drink, throw a ball, or swing a golf club, you rely on the complex, interconnected network of bones, muscles, tendons, and ligaments that make up this joint. You can execute more than a thousand different motions thanks to the shoulder's superior mobility.

Yet the anatomical design that makes this joint so versatile also becomes its greatest vulnerability. The shoulder can move in so many directions because it is a shallow ball-and-socket joint, in which the "ball" (the top of the upper arm bone) is larger than the socket it fits into. This puts the shoulder at risk for instability, making it the most commonly dislocated joint in the body. Its unique anatomy also makes it susceptible to sprains and separations, as well as a variety of overuse injuries. Some of the factors that predispose the shoulders to injury are inherited anatomical differences, while others are behavioral, including poor conditioning that can lead to fatigue and poor form while working or participating in sports.

Whether you have an acute (short-term) injury such as a ligament tear from playing sports or doing repetitive actions at work, or you are experiencing chronic (long-term) shoulder pain from arthritis, this report will guide you through the process of diagnosing the source of your pain and mobility loss and finding the most appropriate treatment. The following pages also offer advice on how to find a qualified, experienced physician to address your pain. And you will learn which tests your doctor will use to pinpoint the source of your discomfort. The numerous treatments covered in this report run the gamut from conservative measures like rest and over-the-counter pain relievers—an approach your doctor will likely start with—to the latest, state-of-the-art surgical procedures for repairing and replacing a damaged shoulder joint. Finally, you will learn tips to strengthen and protect your joint to avoid reinjuring it in the future.

Over my 30 years as a practicing orthopedic surgeon, I have treated thousands of people for virtually every condition that affects the shoulder joint. I have seen firsthand how the proper interventions can restore mobility, relieve pain, and return my patients to their previous level of function. I hope this report will serve as your guide through shoulder repair and recovery and help you communicate more effectively with your doctor as you move through the process.

Sincerely,

Jon J.P. Warner, M.D.

Jon J.P. Warner, M.D.
Medical Editor

Why do we get shoulder pain?

The back, hips, and knees monopolize the spotlight when it comes to joint problems, but the shoulders are also prone to injury, overuse, and disease. In fact, the shoulders are surpassed only by the lower back and knees for producing musculoskeletal pain that causes patients to seek medical advice.

There are many ways in which shoulder damage occurs. The shoulder is the third most likely joint—just behind the hips and knees—to be affected by the degenerative disease osteoarthritis. Although the shoulder joint does not bear the brunt of the body's weight, as the knees and hips do, it can suffer a similar loss of cartilage, leading to pain, stiffness, and lost function. Overuse—such as the persistent wear and tear from repetitive motions like hitting a golf ball, swinging a tennis racket, or pulling heavy items off high shelves at work—can lead to tendinitis or bursitis, while poor posture and biomechanics can cause shoulder impingement. Accidents can lead to bone fractures and tendon tears.

Up to 70% of people will experience shoulder pain at some point in their lives. At any given time, an estimated 9% of American adults who report pain point to the shoulder as its source—and up to a quarter of those who complain of shoulder pain have had at least one previous episode, which indicates that the problem is likely to persist or return after treatment. And while any chronic pain is problematic, shoulder pain can be particularly vexing, because it makes it hard to sleep. With knee pain or back pain, you can usually maneuver into a comfortable position. With shoulder pain, it becomes impossible to sleep on your side.

But why is the shoulder so troublesome? The answer comes down to the shoulder's unique structure, the constant demands we place on it throughout the day, and a variety of risk factors. Fortunately, there are remedies for shoulder trouble, as later chapters of this report will discuss.

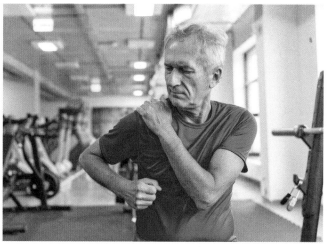

© izusek | Getty Images

The anatomical engineering that affords the shoulder enough range of motion to pitch a softball or scratch your back also gives this joint an inherent instability that makes it more vulnerable to damage.

Shoulder instability

The vulnerability of the shoulder stems in large part from its design. The shoulder is the most mobile joint in the body. It permits an exceptional range of motion—letting you swing your arms forward and backward, extend them out to the side at any angle, raise them above your head, and rotate them inward and outward (see Figure 1, page 3). The arrangement of muscles, tendons, and ligaments allows you to move not just your arms, but the shoulders themselves, scrunching them up around your ears, rolling them forward and backward, and pulling the shoulder blades toward each other.

But that flexibility comes at a price. The anatomical engineering that affords the shoulder enough range of motion to pitch a softball or scratch an itch in the middle of the back also gives this joint an inherent instability that makes it more vulnerable to damage.

The shoulder is one of two ball-and-socket joints in the body; the hip is the other one. But the hip has two features that make it more stable than the shoulder. First, because it is weight-bearing and doesn't require the same range of motion as the shoulder, it is surrounded by a stronger girdle of muscles that help support it. Having a stronger bracing of muscles, tendons, and ligaments in the shoulder would restrict its movement, so there is a fundamental trade-off in the shoulder between stability and function that benefits us, for the most part—until it doesn't.

The other reason the hip is more stable than the shoulder is that the hip has a deeper socket into which the "ball" (the top of the thighbone) is inserted. By contrast, the shoulder has a shallow socket that makes it susceptible to a broader range of problems. And because the shoulder has so many moving parts, an injury to any one of these structures can have a domino effect that leads to significant pain, weakness, and disability.

The shoulder's shallow ball-and-socket structure is in part the heritage of our primate ancestors. Unlike wolves or lions, for example, whose shoulders' main task was to allow walking or running on all fours—basically, moving forward and backward in a single plane—chimpanzee and gorilla shoulders evolved for hanging and swinging. This required greater flexibility and a larger arc of rotation than needed for simple four-footed locomotion.

As humans completed the transition to bipedal movement, the shoulder continued to evolve. Without the demand of having to support the entire weight of the body while hanging from a tree limb, the musculature surrounding the joint slimmed down, thereby allowing an even greater degree of movement. The shape of the shoulder blade also changed, facilitating a broader range of motion—but less strength and stability. And the orientation of the shoulder shifted, with the joint pointing outward rather than forward.

In a groundbreaking paper published in the journal *Nature*, researchers at Harvard and other institutions showed that the combined effect of these changes was that human shoulders developed a unique ability to throw objects at high speed—a skill that likely assisted with both self-defense and hunting, as humans were able to hurl rocks or other projectiles at potential predators and prey. "Some primates, including chimpanzees, throw objects occasionally, but only humans regularly throw projectiles with high speed and accuracy," wrote the scientists. As any sports fan knows, the arm and shoulder can generate baseball pitches or tennis serves that exceed 100 mph.

The next chapter delves into the specifics of shoulder anatomy—explaining the bones, muscles, tendons, and ligaments and how they work together as a whole. There the full complexity of shoulder design becomes clear.

Accidents and other stresses

In a perfect world, we would never stress our shoulders in ways that lead to trouble. But, of course, we do. We take risks; we ski that icy slope and climb that rickety ladder. Falls from a height—such as while horseback riding or bike riding—can cause shoulder sprains and fractures. So can car accidents and even something like tripping on a curb. When you fall on an outstretched arm, a poor landing can send an immediate snap of pain through your shoulder. Dislocations or tears can result from a fall or an intense hit or collision while playing a contact sport such as football or ice hockey.

Injuries are sudden. But problems can also build

Figure 1: The versatile shoulder

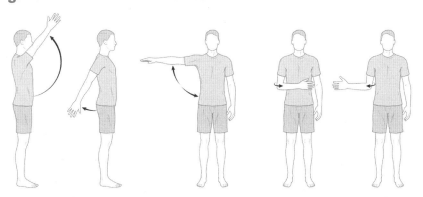

Unlike some joints—such as the knee or finger joints, which are essentially hinges—the shoulder is designed to allow movement in many directions. As a result, we can swing our arms all the way forward and above our heads, push them back behind our bodies, lift them out to the side, and rotate them inward and outward.

up more slowly over time. One of the most common causes of shoulder pain is overuse. Any repeated overhead motion—for example, pitching a softball, serving in tennis, swimming, or casting while fly fishing—can inflame or injure the tendons in a key shoulder structure known as the rotator cuff. The shoulder may have evolved to throw fastballs, but it was never intended to repeat the same motion over and over, hour after hour.

Work-related stresses on the shoulder include not only repetitive movements, such as lifting, but also heavy exertion or even vibrations (such as from a jackhammer or other power tool). But you don't have to have a physically demanding job to suffer shoulder problems from it. If you work in an office, ergonomic factors also play a role in triggering shoulder pain. Poor posture—for example, cradling a phone between your neck and shoulder or sitting on the edge of your chair and hunching over your computer keyboard—can lead to shoulder pain (see "Poor posture and shoulder pain: What's the connection?" on page 24).

Risk factors

A number of factors increase your likelihood of developing shoulder pain, including age, gender, and genes. Even being overweight or smoking can play a role. Some of these factors fall within your control, while others are beyond it.

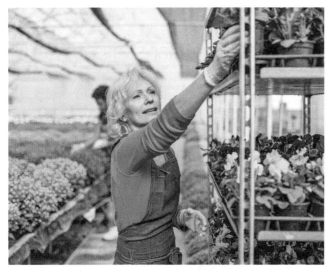

The shoulder is the most versatile joint in the body—and also the most complex, setting it up for a variety of injuries. Repeated overuse, for example, can lead to tendinitis or bursitis.

Genes

Certain shoulder problems seem to run in families. Rotator cuff injuries are more likely to occur not only in siblings, but also in cousins and other more distant relatives. The tendency to injury may be due at least in part to inherited anatomical differences in the shoulder joint. It's also possible that family members tend to share shoulder-straining experiences—for example, if they play the same sports or have the same physically demanding occupation.

Arthritis also has a genetic component. Inherited characteristics in the shape of the acromion (a bony projection on the end of the shoulder blade) and the glenoid cavity (the socket in the shoulder joint) can increase the likelihood of shoulder degeneration and damage.

Age

Your likelihood of developing osteoarthritis increases as you age. Years of playing tennis and golf or engaging in other repetitive activities can cause minor injuries that add up over time, eventually leading to a loss of the cartilage that cushions your shoulder joints. Osteoarthritis and soft tissue conditions, such as rotator cuff injury (see page 16), shoulder impingement syndrome (see page 24), and frozen shoulder (see page 21), are the most common causes of shoulder pain in older adults.

Gender

Women are at higher risk for shoulder pain than men. Their smaller size, coupled with generally weaker muscles, leads to greater shoulder instability. In addition, after a woman spends years playing sports or engaging in repetitive motions at work, her shoulder joints begin to loosen, putting her at increased risk for dislocation. Hormones might play a role in gender-related shoulder differences. Relaxin, the hormone released during pregnancy to ease delivery, does so by relaxing ligaments throughout the body. For these reasons, women are more likely to suffer injuries when they play sports. However, because men participate in sports more over all, they account for a greater proportion of sports-related shoulder injuries.

© AzmanL | Getty Images

Obesity

Extra weight puts added pressure on the joints, and the heavier you are, the more weight your joints have to bear. The knees and hips carry most of this force, but shoulders can be affected, too. Obesity might also contribute to shoulder pain by triggering the release of inflammatory substances. Inflammation activates pain receptors in the area, contributing to shoulder pain.

Other medical conditions

People with certain medical disorders are more likely to develop shoulder pain. These disorders include diabetes, multiple sclerosis, fibromyalgia, and inflammatory forms of arthritis, such as such as rheumatoid arthritis and psoriatic arthritis.

In diabetes, chronic high blood sugar leads to connective tissue damage and inflammation in the shoulders, as well as in other parts of the body. Frozen shoulder and rotator cuff injuries are particularly common in people with diabetes. Although researchers don't know exactly why, it may have to do with impaired blood flow. Another possible culprit is the formation of damaging substances known as advanced glycation end products. These substances—which form when blood sugar is high, and sugar molecules attach abnormally to protein or fat—can make tendons stiff and weak.

Multiple sclerosis causes nerve damage, which leads to pain, weakness, and reduced function throughout the body, including the shoulders. Fibromyalgia is marked by muscle pain and tenderness at various sites, including the neck and shoulders. And inflammatory forms of arthritis produce inflammation in the joints.

Smoking

Along with the many other ill effects of cigarette smoking—among them cancer, heart disease, and lung disease—some studies have linked this harmful habit to shoulder pain, tendon injury, and an increased risk for rotator cuff tears. Smoking promotes inflammation, and it robs the blood of the oxygen needed to heal injuries in the shoulders and elsewhere in the body.

People who smoke tend to have larger rotator cuff tears, and they don't improve as much after rotator cuff surgery as nonsmokers, according to a 2018 study in *BMJ Open Sport & Exercise Medicine.* Another study found that smokers didn't heal well after rotator cuff repair. Nicotine—the active component in tobacco smoke—reduces blood flow to the rotator cuff, an area of the body that already has a limited blood supply. A steady flow of oxygen- and nutrient-rich blood is essential for maintaining a healthy rotator cuff, as well for promoting healing after surgery. ⬗

The anatomy of the shoulder

The shoulder joint is one of the most complex structures in the human body. A feat of anatomical engineering, it is formed by the intersection between three bones—the scapula (shoulder blade), humerus (upper arm bone), and clavicle (collarbone)—together with the many tissues that support the bones and enable them to move smoothly. No fewer than 13 muscles cross the shoulder—large muscles on the outside and smaller ones underneath. Plus there are tendons and ligaments in various layers.

Because the shoulder is multilayered—and includes so many parts—its structure can be hard to understand. This chapter will help.

How joints work

Before delving into shoulder anatomy, a brief overview of joint design in general may be useful. Bones are connected at joints, and it is the arrangement of bones, muscles, ligaments, and tendons in the body that enables you to move. The body contains three basic kinds of joints (see Figure 2, page 7).

Fixed joints, or sutures, are thin bands of fibrous tissue that connect the platelike bones of the skull, allowing the skull to expand and accommodate the growing brain. When brain growth is complete, these fibrous joints disappear as the skull bones fuse.

Cartilaginous joints contain tough cartilage plates. In the pelvis, these joints permit slight movement of the pubic bones and the sacroiliac joint, where the sacrum (part of the spinal column) and pelvis meet. The junctions between the vertebral bones in the spine are also cartilaginous joints; thick discs between the vertebrae accommodate mobility.

Synovial joints are the most mobile. These are found in the shoulders and in other joints that are primarily responsible for your motion, including the elbows, wrists, fingers, hips, knees, ankles, and toes. They take their name from the synovium, a membrane that lines the joint. The synovium produces synovial fluid, which nourishes and lubricates the joints and enables them to be more mobile than cartilaginous joints. Synovial joints are designed for a variety of movements that make possible all manner of activity, from playing tennis to playing the piano. Some—for example, the outermost joints of the fingers—are limited to bending and straightening within a single plane. Others, such as the shoulder, wrist, and hip, are capable of complex movements in multiple planes. Different movements require different configurations of synovial joints. Types of synovial joints include the following:

- **Ball-and-socket joints** (hips and shoulders). In this type of joint, the ball is formed by the head of a long bone—either the femur in the leg or the humerus in the arm. The bone fits into a socket of another bone located in the trunk of the body. These joints are the most mobile, allowing movement in multiple planes.

- **Hinge joints** (elbows, knees, fingers, and toes). In these joints, a protrusion on one bone fits into an indentation in another. Like the hinge on a jewelry box or a gate, these joints allow bending and straightening in a single plane.

- **Pivot joints** (between the two top vertebrae in the neck, and between the radius and humerus at the elbow). In these joints, the head of one bone fits into a ring of connective tissue on another. These joints allow you to turn your head from side to side and to rotate your palm to face up or down while keeping the upper arm still.

- **Gliding joints** (between the breastbone and the ribs, the ribs and spine, and collarbone and shoulder blade). In these joints, two bones meet at flat or slightly curved surfaces and are held together by ligaments (bands of connective tissue) that allow the two surfaces to shift their positions relative to each other.

Features that protect synovial joints

Synovial joints, like machines with moving parts, are vulnerable to friction. If a machine's moving parts come in contact with one another, friction will scratch the surfaces and cause pitting, distortion, and eventually breakage. Two strategies can prevent such friction: applying a lubricant, or inserting a cushion, such as a rubber gasket. Synovial joints are protected in both ways. Following are the joint components that help:

Synovial fluid. Lubrication comes from synovial fluid, a viscous, yellowish, translucent liquid that's produced by the synovium. This fluid not only oils the joint and minimizes friction; it also protects the joint by forming a sticky seal that enables abutting bones to slide freely against each other but resist pulling apart.

Articular cartilage. Cushioning is provided by articular cartilage, a tough and somewhat elastic tissue that covers the ends of bones. Because it's about 75% water, cartilage compresses under pressure (as occurs in the hip with walking or running and in the shoulder with simply raising your arm out to the side) and resumes its original thickness when the force is released, much like a very tough sponge. Because articular cartilage molds to its surroundings, the opposing surfaces of a joint are perfectly matched.

Bursae. It's not just the inside surfaces of joints that are susceptible to damage. Places where tendons and muscles cross over a bone or another muscle are also subject to friction. These sites are protected by bursae, sacs that contain lubricating fluid and act as cushions.

Tendon sheaths. Where tendons are subject to friction, they are also wrapped in protective tissue.

Features that maintain stability in synovial joints

Several things help maintain stability through a joint's range of motion so that the joint can function nor-mally. One is the contour and fit of the joint surfaces themselves. Ligaments and tendons—two forms of connective tissue—also play an important role. The main proteins that make up these tissues are collagens and elastins, which imbue them with tensile strength and elasticity.

Ligaments. Ligaments are tough, slightly elastic, fibrous bands that bind one bone to another. The knee, for example, has four separate ligaments that connect the bones of the upper and lower leg—not only linking them, but also limiting rotation and sideways motion to help stabilize the joint. Ligaments are important for alignment. For example, ligaments on the sides of the finger joints prevent side-to-side bending, while ligaments stretching across the palm keep the fingers from bending too far backward.

Tendons. These are the fibrous cords that attach muscle to bone. Together with muscles, they stabilize joints as well as move them. The best example of

Figure 2: Types of joints

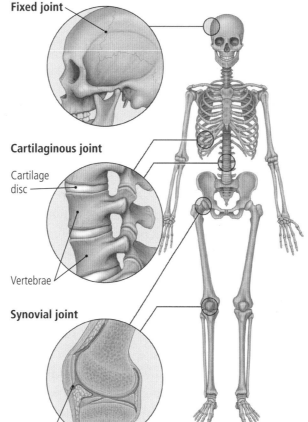

Fixed joint

Cartilaginous joint

Cartilage disc

Vertebrae

Synovial joint

Synovium

There are three basic types of joints.

Fixed joints connect the platelike bones of the skull.

Cartilaginous joints, such as those in the spine and ribs, contain tough cartilage-like plates that bend.

Synovial joints— which are surrounded by a loose fibrous capsule lined with a thin membrane called the synovium—allow the most motion. There are synovial joints throughout the body—for example, in the jaw, shoulders, elbows, wrists, fingers, ankles, hips, knees, and toes.

Figure 3: The shoulder joint

No single illustration can show the anatomy of such a complicated joint as the shoulder, because it contains multiple layers of muscles, tendons, ligaments, bones, and bursae. Furthermore, the shoulder is actually a series of joints working together, two of which are visible in these illustrations. The following views help you peel back the layers to see the areas that may be causing problems.

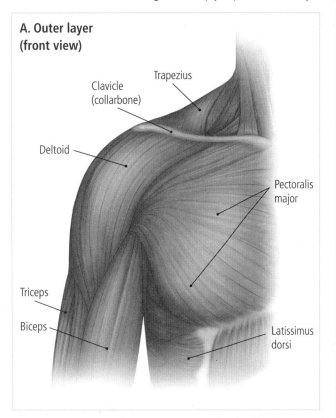

A. Outer layer (front view)

- Trapezius
- Clavicle (collarbone)
- Deltoid
- Pectoralis major
- Triceps
- Biceps
- Latissimus dorsi

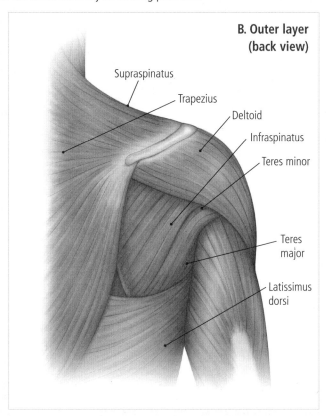

B. Outer layer (back view)

- Supraspinatus
- Trapezius
- Deltoid
- Infraspinatus
- Teres minor
- Teres major
- Latissimus dorsi

Large muscles execute large movements, such as swinging and throwing. The deltoid raises your entire arm, while the pectoralis major (main chest muscle) allows you to lower the arm again and push it out in front of you. In the upper arm, the biceps enables you to bend your arm at the elbow, and the triceps (in back of the arm) extends your arm at the elbow.

In the back, the major muscles include the latissimus dorsi, which pulls the arm down to the side, and the trapezius, which covers most of the upper back and helps move and stabilize the shoulder blade. Between them, you can see a partial view of some of the rotator cuff muscles (go to view D, next page, for more detail).

how this works is in the shoulder, which has a wide range of motion that ligaments would impede. While the large, visible shoulder muscles supply the power to move the shoulder, the small rotator cuff muscles and tendons keep the head of the humerus (upper arm bone) from slipping out of the glenoid cavity, a shallow cuplike indentation in the shoulder blade.

The shoulder joint

The shoulder is the most complicated joint in the human body. Like other synovial joints, the shoulder contains bones, muscles, tendons, and ligaments (see

Figure 3, above). They work together to produce the wide variety of motions that make the shoulder the body's most mobile joint.

Bones of the shoulder

Three bones—the scapula, humerus, and clavicle—connect to form the shoulder.

The humerus (upper arm bone) starts at the elbow and extends to the shoulder. Its bulbous top forms the "ball" in the shoulder's ball-and-socket joint.

The scapula (shoulder blade) is a flat triangular bone that lies on top of the ribs in your upper back.

Continued on page 10

Figure 3: The shoulder joint *continued*

C. Inner layer (front view)

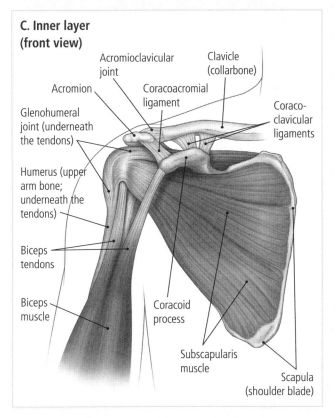

Acromioclavicular joint

Clavicle (collarbone)

Acromion

Coracoacromial ligament

Coraco-clavicular ligaments

Glenohumeral joint (underneath the tendons)

Humerus (upper arm bone; underneath the tendons)

Biceps tendons

Biceps muscle

Coracoid process

Subscapularis muscle

Scapula (shoulder blade)

D. Inner layer (back view)

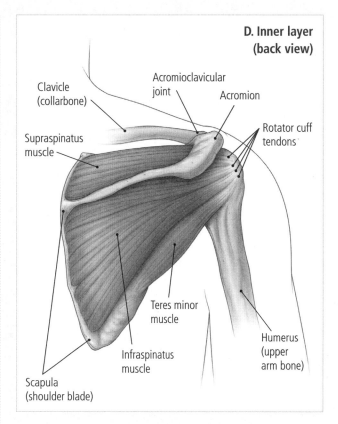

Clavicle (collarbone)

Acromioclavicular joint

Acromion

Rotator cuff tendons

Supraspinatus muscle

Teres minor muscle

Humerus (upper arm bone)

Infraspinatus muscle

Scapula (shoulder blade)

Three important bones—the collarbone (clavicle), upper arm bone (humerus), and shoulder blade (scapula)—converge at the shoulder. The shoulder's main joint, the glenohumeral joint, is formed by the ball at the top of the upper arm bone and the glenoid socket in the shoulder blade, with the coracoclavicular ligaments providing further stabilization on top. (To see beneath the muscles and tendons, go to view E.) The shoulder blade is behind the rib cage (not shown). In this view, you can see the subscapularis, the rotator cuff muscle that lies between the scapula and the rib cage.

Four small muscles—the supraspinatus, infraspinatus, and teres minor (all seen in this view), and the subscapularis (seen in view C)—support and stabilize the shoulder. The tendons of these four muscles connect the shoulder blade to the upper arm bone at the shoulder joint, and together they form the rotator cuff, which gives stability to the shoulder and helps move the humeral head in the socket. The acromion, a bony extension that branches off the main part of the shoulder blade, attaches to the collarbone, providing further stabilization at the acromioclavicular joint.

E. Inside the glenohumeral joint (front view)

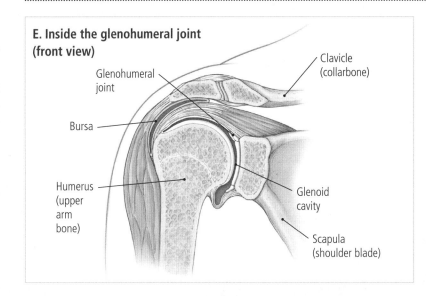

Glenohumeral joint

Clavicle (collarbone)

Bursa

Humerus (upper arm bone)

Glenoid cavity

Scapula (shoulder blade)

Many shoulder injuries involve the shoulder's main joint, the glenohumeral joint, which is formed where the humerus connects with the shoulder socket (called the glenoid, an indentation in the scapula, or shoulder blade). In this view, it becomes clear just how shallow the socket of the glenoid cavity is. Without the ligaments and tendons that hold the humerus in place, it would easily slide out of position. Even with this support, the glenohumeral joint is the most commonly dislocated joint in the body. From this view, you can also see one of the bursae that help prevent friction in the shoulder.

Continued from page 8

You've likely been aware of your shoulder blades for most of your life without realizing that they not only attach to shoulder muscles, but actually form part of the ball-and-socket joint. The socket consists of a slightly hollowed-out area of the scapula called the glenoid cavity (or glenoid socket). However, the socket is too shallow for the ball of the humerus to fit all the way into. Instead, the top of the humerus aligns with the curve and is held in place by ligaments and tendons.

The clavicle (collarbone) is the long horizontal bone that connects your breastbone to the shoulder. It acts to stabilize the scapula relative to the rest of the shoulder and serves as the attachment point for many muscles that help the shoulder joint move. In birds, this bone is very large and strong. That was also the case for our primate ancestors, who swung from trees and thus needed a strong clavicle. Since people don't fly or swing from trees, the human clavicle is smaller. It is also the most commonly fractured bone in the body, since it is often injured when we fall forward and hit the ground.

The clavicle connects to the scapula via two bony projections that branch off the otherwise triangular body of the scapula:

- The acromion reaches from the back of the scapula, extends sideways across the supraspinatus muscle, and goes over the top of the shoulder to the clavicle, where the two bones form the acromioclavicular joint. The joint's name comes from the Greek *akros*, meaning "highest," and *omos*, meaning "shoulder" (see Figure 3, view D, page 9).
- The coracoid process is a small, hooklike structure that extends from the *front* of the scapula and is the attachment point for a series of ligaments that connect the scapula to the clavicle (see Figure 3, view C, page 9). The name coracoid means "shaped like a crow's beak."

The four shoulder joints

The shoulder has one main joint—the ball-and-socket joint to which the arm attaches. But there are three other joints that help stabilize it. Here are all four:

The glenohumeral joint is the main joint of the shoulder, and the one people typically think of as the shoulder joint. It is the region of the shoulder where the ball of the humerus fits into the socket of the scapula (see Figure 3, view E, page 9). The glenohumeral is the most flexible joint in the body. It allows the shoulder to rotate and move in and out, giving it a full range of motion. You use this joint whenever you raise your arm or swing your arm forward or backward. If the ball comes out of the joint, this is called a dislocation.

The acromioclavicular joint (commonly called the AC joint) forms where short, sturdy ligaments connect the clavicle to the acromion at the top of the shoulder (see Figure 3, view D, page 9). This forms a gliding joint that enables you to lift your arms by functioning as a pivot point for movement of the scapula. You use this joint to wave to a friend or lift a pot off a high shelf. An accident such as a fall can cause the two bones to come apart in an injury known as a shoulder separation.

The sternoclavicular joint (not shown) is the saddle-shaped joint that sits at the junction where the clavicle connects with the breastbone (sternum). It allows for movement between the two bones. You use this joint to raise and lower your shoulders—for example, in a shrug. The joint rarely suffers injuries, but a forceful blow to the shoulder sometimes causes the clavicle to dislocate, moving either in front of or behind the breastbone.

The scapulothoracic joint (not shown) is located at the point where the scapula and ribs meet at the back of the torso. Unlike the other shoulder joints, this is not a true synovial joint (that is, connected with ligaments and lined with cartilage and synovial tissue), but rather the place where the ribs and shoulder blade slide past one another. This joint allows for movement between the outer part of the clavicle and the acromion. It enables the up and down, in and out, and rotating movements of the scapula. You use this joint when you shrug your shoulders, punch and retract your fist, or raise your arms above your head.

The rotator cuff, shoulder muscles, and other structures

Like other synovial joints, the shoulder joints are made up of more than just bones. A collection of muscles, ligaments, cartilage, tendons, and other structures support the shoulder, protect it, and help it move. Among these are the crucial rotator cuff muscles (see page 12). Because the socket of the shoulder joint is so shallow—and because the range of movements required is so broad—these additional structures are essential to shoulder function. Collectively, they form what is known as the shoulder girdle.

Cartilage (the smooth material that covers the ends of bones) enables the humerus to move easily and comfortably within the joint. The shoulder contains two types of cartilage, which can both suffer injuries.

- Articular cartilage lines the head of the humerus and the glenoid cavity. It provides a slippery surface for these bones to slide smoothly over one another each time you move your arm. However, it can be damaged by arthritis.
- The labrum is a thick rim of cartilage around the edge of the glenoid cavity that gives the shoulder joint more depth and stability, and helps to prevent the ball from falling out of its socket. Accidents can tear the labrum (a problem known as a labral tear).

The joint capsule is a fibrous sheath that surrounds the glenohumeral joint, as well as the other shoulder joints. The capsule consists of two layers:

- The outer layer is an extension of the ligaments, the fibrous connective tissue that joins the bones.
- The inner, synovial layer contains the synovial membrane, which lubricates the joint, facilitating smooth movement.

The glenohumeral capsule is loose when your arm is at rest at your side. When you move your arm, the capsule and its ligaments act like seat belts and airbags, preventing excess rotation that could damage the joint.

Ligaments (the thick, ropey structures that connect bones to other bones) help stabilize various joints within the shoulder. In the shoulder's main joint, they connect the ball to the socket (that is, the humerus to the glenoid cavity of the scapula). Three of these ligaments—superior, middle, and inferior—work together to prevent the shoulder from dislocating. Ligaments also surround and support the sternoclavicular and acromioclavicular joints.

Tendons (the thick fibers that connect muscles to bones) enable muscles to exert force on bones and move them. With multiple muscles attaching to the shoulder, it is a crowded space, where many tendons converge. For example, the biceps muscle connects to the bones of the shoulder via two biceps tendons (see Figure 3, view C, page 9). Where these attach to the glenoid, they become part of the labrum and help keep the humerus within its socket.

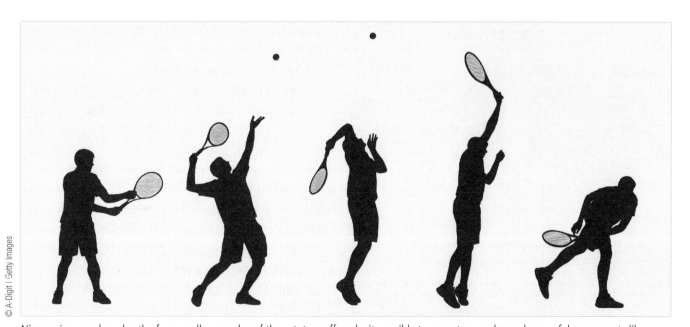

Nine major muscles, plus the four smaller muscles of the rotator cuff, make it possible to execute complex and powerful movements like serving a tennis ball. But the shoulder's large range of motion also makes it subject to instability that can lead to injuries.

© A-Digit | Getty Images

The rotator cuff muscles are the four small muscles of the inner layer of the shoulder (see Figure 3, views C and D, page 9). These small muscles—the supraspinatus, infraspinatus, teres minor, and subscapularis (known collectively as the SITS muscle for the first letter of each of their names)—support the glenohumeral joint. Where their tendons attach to the humerus, they form a fibrous capsule that helps hold the ball in its socket. Together these muscles and their tendons are known as the rotator cuff.

The rotator cuff muscles have many functions. In addition to keeping the ball of the humerus inside the glenoid cavity, they also help rotate the shoulder in many directions. Each one is responsible for a particular type of movement (see Figure 1, page 3):

- The supraspinatus helps to lift the arm out to the side (a movement known as abduction). It is the most likely muscle in the shoulder to tear.
- The infraspinatus enables the arm to rotate sideways from the body (lateral rotation).

Figure 4: Muscles of the neck

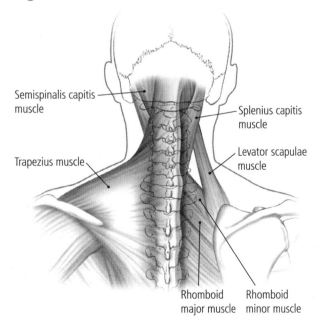

The posterior (rear) neck muscles do the lion's share of work in supporting the weight of your head while tilting and turning. But two of the most important neck muscles—the trapezius (shown only on the left in this illustration) and the levator scapulae (in the deeper muscle layer underneath the trapezius, shown only on the right)—also connect to the shoulders. Also visible here are the rhomboid muscles, which connect the scapula to the spinal column.

- The teres minor also enables the arm to rotate sideways from the body (lateral rotation).
- The subscapularis allows the arm to move toward the body or behind the back (adduction, medial rotation).

Rotator cuff injuries are common. And when people go to physical therapy for their shoulders, it is often the rotator cuff muscles that are the particular focus of the exercises.

Larger muscles of the shoulder's outer layer give the shoulder the strength needed to execute more powerful movements, like swinging a bat.

- The deltoid is the triangular-shaped, bulky muscle at the top of the shoulder. Its main action is to abduct (lift) the arm, but it is also involved with flexion, extension, and lateral rotation (see Figure 1, page 3).
- The pectoralis major is another large, powerful muscle. It starts at the collarbone and connects to the humerus. Contraction of this muscle produces adduction (pulling the arm down to the side) and internal rotation of the arm. You use this muscle whenever you do push-ups.
- The pectoralis minor is a smaller, flat muscle located underneath the pectoralis major. It stabilizes the shoulder blade and lifts the ribcage, among other functions.
- The latissimus dorsi is a thin but wide muscle that stretches across the back. It helps pull the arm down to the side. You use this muscle when doing pull-ups or swimming.
- The trapezius is a broad, flat muscle that creates a diamond-like shape from the base of the neck to the middle of the back (see Figure 4, at left). It attaches to the scapula. You use this muscle to shrug your shoulders, turn your head, and twist your arms.
- The levator scapulae muscle originates in the spinal column of the neck and attaches to the scapula (see Figure 4, at left). It helps to raise and rotate the scapula; for example, when you shrug your shoulders.
- Rhomboids are a pair of muscles (major and minor; see Figure 4, at left) that reach from the spine to the scapula. Their main function is to retract the scapula.
- The serratus anterior muscle is a fan-shaped muscle

that covers the side of the rib cage and inserts into the scapula. It allows for the forward and upward rotation of the arm, which enables you to lift your arms over your head, and it helps stabilize the scapula.

- The teres major is a small muscle that runs along the sides of the scapula. It works together with the latissimus dorsi to adduct and internally rotate the arm, earning it the nickname "lat's little helper."

Bursae are fluid-filled sacs that cushion and prevent friction between bones and other tissues (skin, tendons, muscles). The shoulder joint has six bursae—more than any other joint in the body:

- The subacromial bursa sits between the rotator cuff tendons and the bony acromion. It allows the rotator cuff to move freely when you move your arm. Of the six, it is the one most likely to develop problems.
- The subdeltoid bursa is between the deltoid muscle and the shoulder joint cavity.
- The subcoracoid bursa is between the coracoid process of the scapula and the shoulder joint capsule.
- The infraspinatus bursa is between the infraspinatus tendon and the joint capsule.
- The subcutaneous acromial bursa is above the acromion, just under the skin.

- The subscapular bursa is between the tendon of the subscapularis muscle and the shoulder joint capsule.

Inflammation or irritation of the bursae is called bursitis (see page 14).

How the neck and shoulders interact

The neck and shoulders are separate entities, with, for the most part, separate muscles, joints, and ligaments controlling their respective movements. However, they are close collaborators, and it sometimes is tough to know where neck pain ends and shoulder pain begins.

If you feel an ache in both your neck and shoulders, there's a good chance that the source of the pain is the trapezius muscles (see Figure 4, page 12). The trapezius muscles are true multitaskers. They work with upper back and neck muscles to support your head and neck while collaborating with more than a dozen shoulder muscles to stabilize and move the large triangular shoulder blades. The trapezius muscles are among 30 different muscles that work with key ligaments and tendons to provide movement and support for the entire shoulder. ♥

Common shoulder problems

Given the complexity of shoulder anatomy and the joint's many intersecting parts, it's not surprising that any number of problems can occur that cause pain. Bursae can become inflamed, muscles or tendons can tear, and cartilage and bone can gradually degrade from arthritis. The delicate positioning of the ball in the socket leaves the shoulder vulnerable to instability, and possibly dislocation if subjected to a hard enough blow or fall.

This chapter explores some common causes of shoulder pain and their symptoms. Some conditions are minor enough to treat yourself, while others require a trip to the doctor (see "When to call a doctor," page 15). Note that in some circumstances, shoulder pain originates elsewhere in the body (see "Shoulder pain that isn't caused by a shoulder problem," below left). In some of these instances, shoulder pain can signal a much more serious health issue that requires immediate attention.

Following are the most typical shoulder problems, arranged in order from the most to the least common. Each section starts with a short patient story to give you a better idea of how that problem might occur. (These accounts are composites rather than case reports of individual patients.)

Shoulder pain that isn't caused by a shoulder problem

Pain that you feel in the shoulder does not necessarily come from the shoulder itself. Such pain is called "referred pain," meaning that it has traveled to the shoulder from another location—sometimes from another region of the body entirely. For example, a ruptured spleen can cause pain in the back of the shoulder. Pain from a cervical disc rupture in the neck can radiate to the shoulder. Referred pain may occur when the brain misinterprets which nerve pathways the pain has traveled through.

Watch out for these symptoms, which could indicate a problem unrelated to the shoulder:

- neck pain, numbness and tingling in the arm, weakness (a possible indication of cervical spine disease)

- pain in the center or upper right part of the abdomen, back pain, nausea, vomiting (gallbladder disease)

- pain or tenderness in the upper left side of the abdomen, dizziness (ruptured spleen)

- chest pain or pressure, pain that radiates to the jaw or arms, shortness of breath, nausea, dizziness (heart attack).

It's important to see your doctor for the correct diagnosis, so you can start on the most appropriate treatment. For example, shoulder pain that stems from a cervical disc problem needs to be managed by an orthopedic specialist who treats disorders of the cervical spine.

A heart attack is a medical emergency. If you have shoulder pain along with symptoms like chest pain and pressure, shortness of breath, or nausea, call 911 or go to an emergency room right away.

Bursitis

Sean, a 50-year-old employee at a home improvement company, was responsible for pulling boxes off the warehouse shelves and delivering them to customers at the front of the store. His technique was not ideal, and often the boxes were very heavy. Eventually, he began to notice that his right shoulder—the one he used to lift the boxes—had turned red. The outside of that shoulder ached, and the pain increased whenever he tried to sleep on his right side. He saw his primary care doctor, who diagnosed him with bursitis.

Sean asked his company to temporarily move him to a desk job while his injury healed. He took naproxen (Aleve), an over-the-counter anti-inflammatory drug, a couple of times a day to bring down the swelling and pain. After a couple of weeks, his shoulder still hurt, so his doctor suggested he get a corticosteroid shot. The injection did the trick. Once Sean's shoulder felt well enough, he returned to his old position, but he worked with an occupational therapist to learn the correct lifting techniques to prevent another injury.

Bursae are fluid-filled sacs found in the shoulder, elbow, hip, and other areas of the body. They act as cushions, providing padding and reducing friction between the bones, tendons, and other structures. Like many other shoulder problems, bursitis stems from repetitive or intense motions that put additional pressure on the shoulder. The resulting increase in friction causes one or more of the bursae—most often the subacromial bursa between the rotator cuff tendons and the acromion—to become inflamed and painful. When a loss of flexibility or weakness of the rotator cuff affects shoulder mechanics, the ball of the humerus may move upward, pinching the bursa and causing bursitis (see "Shoulder impingement syndrome," page 24).

Being out of shape or using incorrect form when you play a sport like baseball can also lead to bursitis, since the mechanics of throwing and similar motions require coordinated and conditioned muscles that work properly together. People who develop shoulder pain from repetitive throwing, as well as sports like swimming, often have technique errors and weak core muscles (see "Poor posture and shoulder pain: What's the connection?" on page 24). Certain chronic conditions, such as gout, diabetes, or rheumatoid arthritis, can cause the bursae to swell. Less often, bacteria grow inside a bursa, causing a form of the condition called infected bursitis.

Symptoms of bursitis include

- swelling and redness in the joint
- pain on the outside of your shoulder that may radiate down your arm
- increased pain when you move the shoulder or lie on it.

The first goal in treating bursitis is to bring down inflammation in the bursa, by resting the shoulder, applying ice or heat, and taking nonsteroidal anti-inflammatory drugs (NSAIDs; see "Anti-inflammatories and pain relievers," page 40). Once the swelling has receded and the pain has eased, a few weeks of physical therapy will help recondition the joint and hasten a return to your former routine. If these con-

▶ When to call a doctor

You can generally treat minor shoulder pain related to overuse at home. But more severe or long-term pain, or discomfort that is associated with other symptoms like numbness and weakness, warrants a visit to your primary care provider or an orthopedic specialist.

The following are reasons to call your doctor for shoulder pain:

✔ The pain lasts longer than one week.

✔ The pain interferes with your sleep.

✔ The joint looks deformed.

✔ You can't move the joint without feeling pain.

✔ The pain suddenly increases, or you quickly lose function after an injury such as a fall.

✔ The shoulder is swollen, red, or warm.

servative treatments don't help, a corticosteroid shot into the swollen area may help. Surgery to remove the inflamed bursa and give the rotator cuff more room is a last resort when all other measures fail.

Tendinitis

Kaylee, a junior at a university in southern Florida, is the outside hitter on her school's volleyball team. During a competitive season, with the team striving to reach the No. 1 slot in its division, Kaylee put a lot of power into each hit, but she didn't always use proper form. About halfway through the season, she started complaining to her coach of pain in her shoulder each time she practiced or played. The coach suspected tendinitis, and he suggested she take some time off from practice to allow her injury to heal before the division playoffs. A doctor confirmed the diagnosis and prescribed physical therapy.

Kaylee eased back into her practices slowly, with the help of physical therapy to improve her range of motion, but she wasn't able to put much power into her game. Although she didn't recover enough by playoff time to participate, her coach and physical therapist assured her that with continual gradual exercise, she'd be fully ready to play by the beginning of the following season.

Tendinitis is inflammation of the tendons, the thick cords that connect the ends of muscles to bones, enabling you to move the bones. In the shoulder, tendons help move both the arm and the shoulder itself, and the rotator cuff tendons perform the additional task of helping to stabilize the shoulder.

Tendinitis can affect the rotator cuff tendons as well as the biceps tendons. Symptoms in the shoulder include

- pain in your shoulder, especially when you lift your arm or lie on the affected side
- difficulty holding your arm out to the side or in front of your body
- a clicking, catching, or crunching noise when you move your arm.

Like bursitis, tendinitis results from repetitive stress while playing sports such as tennis, golf, baseball, or swimming. Poor technique while engaging in these sports can put excess pressure on the tendons, hastening injury. Another cause of tendinitis is repeated overhead motions, for example while working on an assembly line or using an overhead pressing machine. In some cases, the condition results from a direct hit to the shoulder or from falling on an outstretched arm.

As with many other shoulder conditions, treatment involves reducing inflammation, which can be accomplished with a combination of rest, NSAIDs (see "Anti-inflammatories and pain relievers," page 40), physical therapy, and sometimes a corticosteroid injection.

Rotator cuff injury

Bob, a 45-year-old marketing executive, took over as pitcher for his company's baseball team. The team practiced three nights a week throughout the spring season and played against other local teams on Saturday afternoons. In his quest to lead his team to a championship, Bob began practicing every night and pitching each game with greater intensity. After a couple of months, he developed pain and tenderness in his right shoulder. It hurt to lift his right arm or to sleep on his right side. Bob saw an orthopedic specialist, who diagnosed him with a rotator cuff tear.

The doctor advised him to sit out baseball practices and games for a while and take nonsteroidal anti-inflammatory medicines to relieve pain and bring

down swelling. Once the pain subsided, Bob's doctor prescribed physical therapy to help him regain strength in the affected shoulder. After three months of therapy, Bob's shoulder was stronger and pain-free. His therapist taught him throwing strategies to avoid reinjuring his shoulder and urged him to limit the number of pitches he throws during practices. Bob was grateful that his injury could be resolved with physical therapy, as he'd heard about more serious cases that required surgery.

The rotator cuff is a group of muscles and tendons that surround the shoulder joint and help to hold it in place (see "Rotator cuff muscles," page 12, and Figure 3, view D, page 9). Injuring your shoulder—for example, by lifting a heavy object or falling on an outstretched arm—can cause a sudden tear in this structure. More commonly, though, rotator cuff injuries are the result of a gradual degenerative process that weakens the tissue to the point where it rips.

Rotator cuff injuries are quite common. It's hard to pinpoint exact numbers, because many of these injuries produce no symptoms or only minimal symptoms, but in imaging studies, 54% of people over age 60 and 65% of people over age 70 show signs of rotator cuff damage. The supraspinatus is the rotator cuff muscle that's most prone to injury. Often, small tears develop over time in the rotator cuff tendons, particularly in the dominant arm.

Being over age 40 is one of the biggest risk factors for rotator cuff injuries. Years of use cause wear and tear that weakens the rotator cuff tendons. "Weekend warriors" who regularly play sports like baseball or tennis are also vulnerable to these injuries, as are people who work in jobs that involve repetitive arm motions or heavy lifting. The propensity for rotator cuff tears also has a genetic component, as these injuries tend to run in families.

Symptoms of a rotator cuff injury include
- aching or pain in the shoulder
- pain when you lift your arm
- difficulty sleeping on the affected side
- weakness in the arm, usually sudden
- reduced movement in the arm, usually because of both pain and weakness.

Conservative treatments such as rest, ice, over-the-counter pain relievers, physical therapy, and activ-

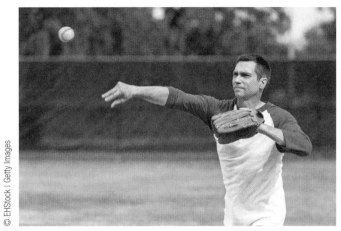

Office workers who regularly play sports like baseball or tennis on the weekends are vulnerable to rotator cuff injuries. These injuries are quite common, affecting up to 40% of people at some point.

ity modification are often enough to treat a rotator cuff injury. A corticosteroid injection into the shoulder can help bring down inflammation and ease pain, but doctors recommend limiting the number of injections you get to no more than four a year. Too many of these shots can weaken the rotator cuff tendon.

For more severe tears that don't readily heal, surgery may be necessary. The tendon can be repaired with an open procedure or arthroscopically (through small incisions). Very significant tears may require shoulder replacement surgery (see "Surgery," page 43).

Biceps tendon tears

Bob, a 50-year-old mechanic, received a delivery of tires at his shop. Since none of his assistants was available to help, he started to carry the tires into the garage himself. As soon as he lifted the first tire, he felt a pop in his shoulder, along with an intense pain. The next day Bob visited an urgent care center, where the doctor told him he had a biceps tendon tear.

Fortunately, Bob hadn't torn his rotator cuff, so he was able to rely on nonsurgical treatments. He took a break from the heavy lifting, letting his assistants take over. Every few hours, Bob held an ice pack to the injured shoulder. He took ibuprofen (Advil) whenever the pain became too uncomfortable. Within five weeks he felt much better, but his doctor cautioned him to avoid lifting anything heavy for a few months to prevent him from reinjuring the biceps tendon.

Your biceps muscle is the strong muscle in the front of your arm that you use to bend your elbow or curl a weight toward your shoulder while weightlifting. It's the same muscle you would flex if someone were to say, "Show me your muscles."

Two tendons attach your biceps to your shoulder. The longer one attaches to the top of the glenoid, or shoulder socket. The shorter one attaches to the coracoid process on the shoulder blade (see Figure 3, view C, page 9). The longer one is the one you are more likely to damage with a traumatic injury, or from years of overusing it while working or playing sports.

Every year, about two out of every 100,000 people tear a biceps tendon—and the vast majority are men. Most biceps tendon tears affect people in their 40s through 60s, although younger people can develop this injury if they lift heavy weights or play a high-contact sport like football. Smoking and the use of steroid medicines can also weaken this tendon and make it more likely to tear.

Damage that occurs over a period of years can cause the biceps tendon to slowly fray, much like a rope that has been pulled for a long period of time. An injury can cause an immediate tear, ripping the tendon away from the shoulder bone.

Symptoms of a biceps tendon tear include
- pain in the upper arm and shoulder
- a popping noise
- weakness in the shoulder
- a bulge in the upper arm above the elbow called a "Popeye muscle" because it resembles the cartoon character's short, wide muscles.

Most biceps tendon tears are easily treatable with ice, rest, NSAIDs (see "Anti-inflammatories and pain relievers," page 40), and physical therapy. Surgery is rarely needed, except for athletes who need to fully recover their strength in order to get back on the field.

Shoulder joint instability and dislocation

Shelley, a 25-year-old registered nurse, took part in a tennis clinic while visiting a resort in Arizona. The tennis pro encouraged her to put more energy into her serve. She threw the tennis ball high into the air with

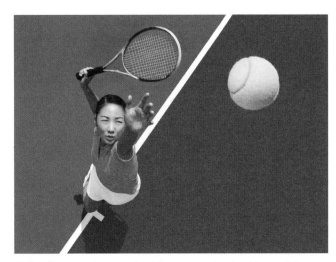

Ordinarily, a tennis serve should not cause the shoulder to dislocate. But repetitive movements can stretch out the shoulder ligaments to the point where they can no longer support the joint.

© nycshooter | Getty Images

her left arm and swung the racket with all the force she could summon from her right shoulder. As soon as the racket hit the ball, she felt a pop in her shoulder, followed by intense pain. A large lump arose from the top of her right shoulder. Fortunately, the tennis pro recognized her injury as a dislocation, and he had the medical training needed to pop her shoulder joint back into place before driving her to a local hospital. The emergency room doctor sent her home with a sling, cautioning her to wear it and avoid tennis and other activities for a few weeks. Once the pain and swelling improved, she began doing the gentle exercises her doctor had recommended. She also worked with a physical therapist to learn safer serving techniques for future tennis outings.

The same anatomical design that gives the shoulder its flexibility also makes it subject to dislocation, when the shallowness of the shoulder socket allows the ball of the upper arm bone to pop out of the socket. One of two terms may apply:

- When the ball comes all the way out of the socket, that's called a dislocation (see Figure 5, page 19).
- When the ball slips only partly out of its socket, doctors refer to the injury as a subluxation.

Dislocation can happen in a few different ways. Repetitive movements can stretch out the shoulder ligaments to the point where they can no longer support the shoulder joint. Swimmers, as well as tennis and volleyball players, are at risk for repetitive strain injuries that lead to dislocations.

Alternatively, a traumatic injury, such as a powerful hit to the shoulder or a fall, can rip the head of the upper arm bone out of the socket. Such an injury may also damage the glenoid bone and tear the labrum (the cartilage rim around the edge of the glenoid cavity) as well as ligaments in the front of the shoulder.

A small number of people with a genetic tendency to have looser-than-normal joints can dislocate a shoulder with only a minor injury or no trauma at all. While most shoulder dislocations involve the ball popping out of the front of the socket, in people with this genetic tendency, the ball can dislocate out of the front, back, or bottom of the socket. This is referred to as multidirectional instability.

Whatever the cause of a shoulder dislocation, symptoms may include

- intense pain
- inability to move the joint
- a shoulder that appears deformed or out of place
- swelling
- bruising
- numbness, weakness, or tingling near the injury.

Once a shoulder has dislocated and the ligaments, muscles, and other structures around the joint have been damaged, they may no longer provide adequate support for the joint. As a result, the shoulder can become chronically unstable and prone to additional injuries. Among people who experience a shoulder dislocation, about one in five will have a second dislocation, and one in 10 will have a third, according to a 2018 study in the *Journal of Shoulder and Elbow Surgery*. The average time to a repeat dislocation is approximately one year.

Symptoms of chronic shoulder instability include

- repeated shoulder dislocations
- pain in the shoulder
- a feeling that the shoulder is always loose
- decreased movement in the shoulder joint.

It is often easy to fix a dislocated shoulder joint with a procedure called a closed reduction, in which gentle traction allows the muscles of the shoulder to relax to the point where the ball can slip back into place. An experienced coach or trainer can sometimes perform a closed reduction, but ideally, you will want to have a doctor perform the procedure at a hospital, because some methods can be very painful. At a medical facility you will get anesthesia, which may involve an injection into the shoulder or medications to keep you comfortable and relaxed. Also, doing this procedure incorrectly could damage the shoulder further and contribute to future instability.

Doctors can use several different approaches to put a dislocated shoulder ball back into its socket. For example, the doctor might slowly pull your arm away from your body into a 90° angle, and then slowly rotate it outward to 90°. This movement relaxes the muscles of the rotator cuff, allowing the humerus to move back into the glenoid socket.

After a reduction, your doctor will usually recommend that you keep your arm immobilized in a sling for a few weeks to give the shoulder a chance to recover. To treat soreness, hold ice to the affected shoulder three or four times a day. Once the pain and swelling go down, you'll likely see a physical therapist to learn exercises for strengthening the shoulder muscles and rebuilding your range of motion. Your doctor may request an MRI or CT scan to see how you are healing.

Arthritis and problems that can cause arthritis

Bettie, a 70-year-old grandmother, started to feel pain in the front of her left shoulder. The shoulder became so sore and stiff that it was hard for her to lift her arm to wave to a friend or reach up to turn off her bedroom light. The continuing discomfort forced her to skip her weekly golf game. Whenever Bettie moved her arm, she heard a clicking or grinding noise. Her primary care doctor took an x-ray of her left shoulder and determined that she had osteoarthritis.

Bettie tried to manage the pain and stiffness by applying a heating pad several times a day and taking over-the-counter pain relievers. She also started on a physical therapy program and began taking twice-weekly gentle yoga classes to keep her shoulder joint mobile. After six months on these treatments with no real improvement, she opted for a total shoulder joint replacement. Her recovery took several months, but today her pain has improved significantly, and she's able to play golf again.

Arthritis is one of the most common and most debilitating afflictions among older adults. It is characterized by joint inflammation, which may be caused by a degenerative process, an autoimmune disease, or an injury. When arthritis strikes, it results in painful, stiff, swollen joints that are difficult to move.

Arthritis can affect any joint in the body, including the hips, knees, and wrists. In the shoulder, it causes inflammation in the acromioclavicular and glenohumeral joints.

Symptoms of shoulder arthritis include
- aches or pain in part or all of the shoulder that may worsen with activity or over time
- stiffness
- swelling in the joint

Figure 5: A normal vs. a dislocated shoulder

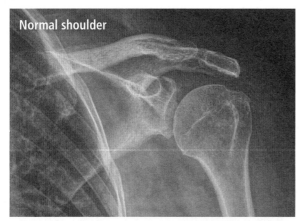

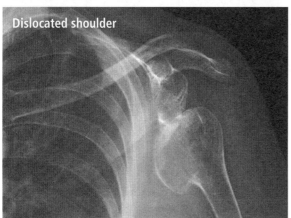

Under normal conditions, the head of the humerus (ball) sits inside the glenoid cavity (socket). In a dislocation, the ball moves completely out of the socket, causing pain, deformity, and restricted movement.

Images: Dr. Jon J.P. Warner, Harvard Medical School.

- limited range of motion in the shoulder
- a cracking or clicking sound when you move your shoulder.

Although osteoarthritis is the best known type of arthritis, it is not the only one that can affect the shoulder. Following are the most common types.

Osteoarthritis

Osteoarthritis is the wear-and-tear form of arthritis that affects more than 30 million Americans, or nearly a third of people over age 60. Its degenerative nature makes it more likely to set in after age 50. Years of throwing, lifting, and engaging in other shoulder motions can cause minor injuries that add up over time, leading to the gradual erosion of the cartilage that protects the bones of the shoulder joints. Normally, the pad of cartilage between the bones creates a space of about 3 millimeters within the joint. In an arthritic joint, this space is narrowed. Without protection from cartilage, the bones of the shoulder joint rub against one another, causing pain, stiffness, and swelling. Arthritis also thickens and scars the joint capsule, which restricts movement even more.

Although osteoarthritis does not affect the shoulder joint as often as it does the hip or knee, shoulder osteoarthritis is still relatively common. And while the shoulder is not a weight-bearing joint, arthritis there can eventually cause enough pain and constriction of movement to become debilitating. Compared with the 900,000 people each year who have a knee or hip replacement, only 53,000 have a shoulder replaced. However, that number is growing at a rate of about 8% annually, which is two to three times faster than that of hip and knee surgery.

The initial treatment for osteoarthritis consists of activity modification, physical therapy, heat or cold, and NSAIDs (see "Anti-inflammatories and pain relievers," page 40). Corticosteroid injections can reduce inflammation and pain temporarily. If these measures don't help, you may need surgery to replace the damaged joint (see "Total shoulder replacement," page 48).

Secondary osteoarthritis

Osteoarthritis can be primary (with no known cause other than aging) or secondary (the result of another identifiable trigger or risk factor). Following are some causes of secondary osteoarthritis in the shoulder.

Trauma. Post-traumatic arthritis is a type of osteoarthritis that results from a dislocation, fracture, or other injury to the shoulder joint—most often, the result of a car accident, sports-related injury, or fall. The injury damages cartilage in the joint and causes it to degenerate more quickly than usual into osteoarthritis. This type of arthritis accounts for about 12% of all osteoarthritis cases. Treatment is similar to that for primary osteoarthritis, including exercise, NSAIDs (see "Anti-inflammatories and pain relievers," page 40), and corticosteroid injections. Surgery is recommended when these interventions are no longer effective.

Rotator cuff tear. Rotator cuff tear arthropathy is a form of arthritis that results from a combination of degeneration and a rotator cuff injury. Normally, the rotator cuff keeps the arm bone stable and tethered in its socket, but a rotator cuff tear—one of the most common injuries to the shoulder—can compromise the strength and stability of the shoulder. The head of the arm bone is then able to drift free and rub against the acromion. Degeneration of cartilage in the shoulder joint, along with the friction of bone rubbing against bone, leads to stiffness, weakness, and difficulty moving the arm. Surgery may be necessary to treat the problem. Because a traditional shoulder replacement requires a healthy rotator cuff, doctors instead perform a reverse total shoulder replacement (see page 48), which alters shoulder mechanics in a way that takes pressure off the injured rotator cuff.

Avascular necrosis. Like all other tissues in the body, bones need oxygen-rich blood to function. A fracture or other injury that disrupts blood flow to the shoulder can cause the bone to die (become necrotic)—a condition known as avascular necrosis, or osteonecrosis. When bone dies, the body tries to heal the damage. It produces cells called osteoclasts to remove dead bone, and cells called osteoblasts to lay down new, healthy bone. Problems arise when osteoclasts dispose of dead bone faster than the body can replace it. The bones become weak, brittle, and vulnerable to collapse. The loss of support underneath the cartilage causes the smooth surface of the ball to give way. This leads to an irregular surface and wear and tear in the joint. Ultimately, arthritis develops.

Treatments for avascular necrosis can range from NSAIDs (see "Anti-inflammatories and pain relievers," page 40) and rest, to blood thinners or osteoporosis drugs to slow the progression of bone damage. Surgery may eventually be needed. Surgical options include a bone transplant—which replaces the damaged piece of bone with a healthy piece of bone taken from another part of your body—or a joint replacement.

Rheumatoid arthritis

Rheumatoid arthritis is an autoimmune disease. The immune system, which is normally responsible for fighting off viruses, bacteria, and other infectious organisms, in this case mistakenly attacks the body—specifically the synovium, the lubricating membrane that lines the joints. This attack inflames the synovium and damages cartilage and bone in the shoulder, as well as in other joints around the body. The resulting damage leads to pain, swelling, and reduced movement. Rheumatoid arthritis is a symmetrical disease, meaning that it affects both shoulders, whereas osteoarthritis may only affect one shoulder.

Treatment for rheumatoid arthritis involves disease-modifying antirheumatic drugs (DMARDs) such as hydroxychloroquine (Plaquenil), methotrexate (Trexall), and sulfasalazine (Azulfidine). Unlike treatments that merely address symptoms, these medications actually slow the disease process to prevent further joint damage. A newer group of DMARDs known as biologic drugs target the specific parts of the immune system that cause the inflammation responsible for joint damage. Biologics include drugs like abatacept (Orencia), adalimumab (Humira), etanercept (Enbrel), and rituximab (Rituxan). Treatment with drugs is now much more effective at reducing the degenerative process than in years past, so fewer people ultimately need surgery. If surgery is required, the results are similar to those of osteoarthritis patients.

Figure 6: Frozen shoulder

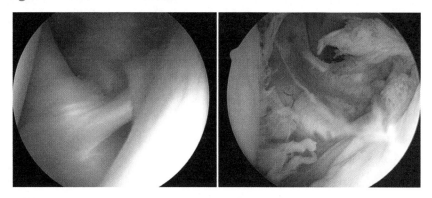

In a normal shoulder (left), the shoulder capsule appears white and thin. With a frozen shoulder (right), the capsule lining is thickened and red from inflammation.
Image: Reproduced with permission from OrthoInfo.
© *American Academy of Orthopaedic Surgeons. http://orthoinfo.aaos.org.*

Frozen shoulder (adhesive capsulitis)

Eloise, a 45-year-old nursing home employee, fell and dislocated her shoulder. She recovered from the fall, but eventually her shoulder stiffened to the point where she could barely move it. It became impossible for her to lift patients at work, or even to get dressed and brush her hair in the morning. She worried that she would lose her job. An orthopedic specialist diagnosed her with frozen shoulder.

Taking over-the-counter pain relievers and doing the exercises her physical therapist prescribed every day improved her movement to the point where daily activities became doable again. Yet her shoulder was still somewhat stiff, making it difficult for Eloise to do her job. Her doctor said a complete recovery could take a year or more, and he gave her the option of having arthroscopic surgery to speed her recovery. She decided to wait, but kept surgery on the back burner as an option.

Frozen shoulder occurs when inflammation and scar tissue invade the shoulder joint (see Figure 6, above). It's believed to be a form of autoimmune disease in which the body overreacts to a minimal injury and then cells in the joint release inflammatory chemicals that cause pain. Ultimately the cells in the joint capsule create scar tissue, which produces a stiff shoulder.

Symptoms of a frozen shoulder include
- stiffness that worsens at first, but gradually begins to improve over time

• dull, aching pain that increases as the disease progresses, and may worsen when you move your arm.

Frozen shoulder affects between 2% and 5% of people over all. Although the exact cause of frozen shoulder isn't clear, it is more common in people with conditions like diabetes, Parkinson's disease, and thyroid disease. Frozen shoulder can also develop after the shoulder has been immobilized for a long period of time—for example, following an injury, a stroke, or surgery. It is more common in women than men.

Frozen shoulder typically progresses through three stages, although the duration of each stage varies from person to person.

Stage 1: Freezing. The shoulder becomes inflamed and the shoulder capsule progressively shrinks, leading to increasing pain and stiffness. This stage can last from two to nine months.

Stage 2: Frozen. The shoulder remains stiff, limiting range of motion. However, the pain begins to recede. This stage lasts from four to six months.

Stage 3: Thaw. The stiffness improves, and you gradually gain more motion in the shoulder. Most of the time the condition gets better on its own, yet it can take between six months and two years to fully regain movement and function in the affected shoulder.

The typical treatment involves physical therapy, along with medication to manage pain and inflammation. However, there is controversy about the role of physical therapy. Too much stretching can worsen the condition, while too little will allow it to continue. This makes it crucial to find the right balance. Often, physical therapists will start with stretches that are very gentle and brief (one to five seconds), and then slowly progress to muscle strengthening and mobility exercises as the shoulder condition improves. In addition to therapy sessions, people should stretch on their own at home to speed healing.

Separated shoulder (shoulder sprain)

Jim, a 42-year-old accountant, plays ice hockey on a men's recreational team in his New England town. His league had always played aggressively, but one weekend, a player from the other team slammed Jim hard into the boards. His shoulder swelled up. The pain was

Shoulder strains

Often confused with a sprain, a shoulder strain affects different structures. While a sprain involves damage to ligaments, a strain occurs when a shoulder muscle or tendon is stretched beyond its limit or tears. This can happen from using poor form, such as when you hunch over a computer, or from carrying a heavy item like a backpack on one shoulder. Repetitive motions in sports such as swimming or tennis can also strain the structures in the shoulder. A shoulder strain is treated in essentially the same way as a sprain—with anti-inflammatory drugs, cold, and physical therapy. Surgery is rarely needed, unless the pain persists and these treatments are ineffective.

so intense that he could barely raise his arm to brush his teeth or comb his hair. He went to the hospital, where the orthopedic doctor on call diagnosed him with a grade 2 shoulder separation. He was put on a regimen of ice and prescription anti-inflammatories to relieve pain and swelling, and advised to wear a sling for two weeks. Once the sling came off, Jim's shoulder felt much better, but he had to sit out ice hockey practice for another four weeks to give the sprain time to fully heal.

A separated shoulder, also known as a shoulder sprain, is an injury to the acromioclavicular (AC) joint. Separation is different from dislocation (see "Shoulder joint instability and dislocation," page 17), another form of shoulder instability that involves the glenohumeral joint—and also different from a shoulder strain (see above).

The AC joint sits at the top of the shoulder, at the point where the collarbone (clavicle) meets the bony projection called the acromion atop the shoulder blade. The acromioclavicular ligament and coracoclavicular ligaments hold the collarbone to the shoulder blade and stabilize the shoulder. These ligaments are tough, and it takes a lot of force to tear them.

To have a shoulder separation, you need to sustain a relatively hard blow to the shoulder; for example, during a car accident or from a tackle in a contact sport such as football or rugby. A hard enough hit can stretch or tear these ligaments, causing the bones of the AC joint to separate.

Doctors divide shoulder sprains into grades based on how much damage the ligaments have sustained and the degree of separation between the collarbone and acromion:

- Grade 1: The ligaments of the AC joint stretch but they don't tear.
- Grade 2: The ligaments tear, causing pain and swelling.
- Grade 3: Tears in the ligaments cause the collarbone to dislocate.
- Grades 4, 5, and 6: Ligaments in the AC tear, the AC joint separates, and muscles detach from the collarbone. Increasing grades mean that the collarbone is pushed even farther from its normal position and the shoulder is more deformed.

Symptoms of a separated shoulder include
- pain in the shoulder
- weakness in the shoulder or arm
- bruising
- swelling
- limited movement in that arm
- a bump at the top of the shoulder
- a feeling like the shoulder joint is unstable.

The term "separated shoulder" makes this injury seem much more dire than it actually is. With a combination of ice, rest, NSAIDs (see "Anti-inflammatories and pain relievers," page 40), and physical therapy, most people find relief from their pain within a couple of weeks. However, it can take six weeks or more to fully return to sports and other activities that rely heavily on the shoulder. If pain persists despite more conservative treatments, surgery to reconstruct the joint is an option.

Fractures (broken bones)

Judy, a 56-year-old vice principal at a high school in the Midwest, liked to spend her weekends horseback riding in the countryside. One spring morning, she was riding through the woods, when the movement of a small animal in the brush caused her horse to startle and rear up. Judy was thrown from the horse, landing directly on her right shoulder. She had severe pain in her right arm, as well as a large bruise and a lump on that shoulder. Her husband drove her to a nearby hospital, where an x-ray revealed a proximal humerus fracture—a broken upper arm bone.

The doctor said she was lucky that the bone was minimally displaced; in other words, it had shifted only slightly out of position at the point of the fracture. That meant Judy could avoid surgery. She had to wear a sling to keep the shoulder immobile and do gentle range-of-motion exercises with a physical therapist. Her doctor checked her six weeks later, and found that the shoulder had healed sufficiently to let her take off the sling. Judy continued to work with her physical therapist, who gradually introduced exercises to help her regain strength in the injured shoulder.

A major blow to the shoulder can cause the collarbone, the shoulder blade, or the top of the upper arm bone (proximal humerus) to fracture—meaning that it forms a crack or break. In severe cases, the bone can break into two or more pieces.

The collarbone is the most likely bone in the shoulder area to break during a fall. It can also fracture as the result of a car or motorcycle accident. Proximal humerus fractures are more common in older adults. Osteoporosis, which occurs more frequently with age, can leave the bones porous and weak enough to break as the result of a fall or a blow to the shoulder. About 85% of all proximal humerus fractures affect people older than 50. Because the shoulder blade is cushioned by the chest, it is most likely to fracture from a high-energy trauma, such as a motor vehicle accident.

Symptoms of a shoulder fracture include
- pain
- swelling
- bruising
- a bump at the fracture site
- difficulty moving the arm
- a grinding sound when you move the arm.

Most proximal humerus fractures—about 80%—are treated conservatively with rest, immobilization in a sling, and physical therapy. The degree of separation in the bone will determine which treatment is recommended. Fractures in which the bones remain aligned (nondisplaced) or have only shifted position slightly (minimally displaced) should heal with these treatments. Bones that have moved position significantly (displaced) likely won't heal well enough to allow normal joint movement in the future. These fractures need to be treated surgically (see "ORIF fracture repair surgery," page 48). ◗

Poor posture and shoulder pain: What's the connection?

Do you hunch over your computer all day at work? Do you slump down in your chair while watching television? Poor posture is increasingly common among Americans. As technology has changed the way we work and interact, our necks, shoulders, and backs have paid the price. Poor posture is a known contributor to back and shoulder pain.

Poor posture changes the position of various shoulder structures in relation to one another. This repositioning alters basic shoulder mechanics, making them less efficient and setting you up for a problem known as shoulder impingement syndrome, which in turn can lead to other problems such as bursitis and tendinitis. Some basic posture checks and simple exercises to improve posture can help.

Shoulder impingement syndrome

In shoulder impingement syndrome, tendons do not have enough space to move properly. Remember that many tendons converge in the narrow space beneath the acromion (the bony, roof-like structure linking the shoulder blade and collarbone). When you raise your arm, this space narrows further, and the acromion can rub against (impinge on) the tendons or bursa—specifically, the rotator cuff tendons and the subacromial bursa.

Constant irritation inflames the tendons and bursa, causing rotator cuff tendinitis, shoulder bursitis, or both. Lying on the affected side becomes painful. Certain movements, such as raising your arm or rotating it inward, also cause pain. Pushed to the extreme, impingement can make even simple things like brushing your hair or dressing yourself difficult, if not impossible. Ultimately, if shoulder impingement is not treated, it can produce enough wear on the tendons and bursa that you develop a rotator cuff tear.

Poor posture is not the only cause of shoulder impingement. Repetitive overhead movements are often responsible. For this reason, shoulder impingement is sometimes called "swimmer's shoulder," although it is hardly limited to swimmers—tennis and basketball players, along with construction workers and housepainters, are also frequent sufferers. People who continually reach up to high shelves are also vulnerable. Additional causes include osteoarthritis and compression resulting from a fall. But poor posture can both cause pain in the first place and make shoulder pain from any of these other causes worse.

If you have shoulder impingement syndrome, the doctor will usually begin by prescribing nonsteroidal anti-inflammatory drugs (NSAIDs) to bring down the swelling. In extreme cases, an injection of corticosteroids in the shoulder may help. But at the same time, don't be surprised if you receive a referral to a physical therapist. While the medications can relieve short-term pain, the work you do with your physical therapist could be the most effective treatment you receive in the long run, because it addresses the cause of the problem, not just the symptoms.

Posture and shoulder mechanics

The problem with poor posture isn't just that it narrows the subacromial space, but that it also affects basic shoulder mechanics. It changes the positioning of the shoulder blade and the arm. This in turn reduces the efficiency of your shoulder muscles as they attempt to move your arm.

A simple test illustrates how dramatically posture affects shoulder function. Sit in a slouched position and raise your arm out to the side as high as possible. Now try the same motion while sitting up straight. The movement when you straighten up is longer and more fluid—not to mention less painful. That's because when you slouch, your shoulder blade angles downward, blocking the ball from fully rotating in the shoulder socket. When you have good posture, the shoulder blade points upward, giving the shoulder ball total freedom to move.

These are some of the most common postural mistakes that can affect the shoulder:

- perching on the edge of your chair, bending your head forward, and rounding your shoulders
- leaning your head and neck forward and flattening your back while standing
- slouching over a tablet or smartphone (known as "text neck")
- standing with your weight on one leg
- sticking out your chin while trying to look up at your computer monitor
- rounding your shoulders (known as "Mom posture")
- walking with your shoulders held forward and your upper back rounded
- carrying heavy items like a backpack or purse on one shoulder.

Practice good posture

The goal of posture work is to improve your posture not just when you're sitting in front of the computer, but throughout your day. Proper alignment whenever you sit or stand will protect your shoulders, neck, and back from extra strain. But what constitutes good posture? When told to stand up straight, people often thrust out their chest and put an unnatural arch in their lower back. This is not good posture.

Instead, try the following. Whenever you stand up, imagine that someone is pulling on a string that goes from your feet to your head and stretches all the way to the ceiling. Your head and neck should be straight. Your shoulders should be directly over your hips, set slightly back but relaxed. Your chest should be a little bit forward. You should have what's known as a neutral spine, which takes the gentle curves of the spine into account, but is not flexed or arched. Keep your feet about hip-distance apart, with your weight balanced equally between them and your knees slightly bent. Pull in your belly.

If you work at a desk for a good portion of the day, the position of your chair and computer monitor can contribute to poor form. Making a few adjustments will reduce the strain on both your back and shoulders (see Figure 7, below).

Figure 7: Proper sitting form

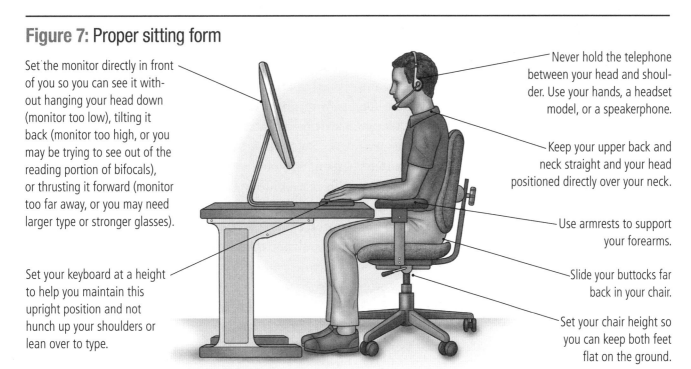

Set the monitor directly in front of you so you can see it without hanging your head down (monitor too low), tilting it back (monitor too high, or you may be trying to see out of the reading portion of bifocals), or thrusting it forward (monitor too far away, or you may need larger type or stronger glasses).

Set your keyboard at a height to help you maintain this upright position and not hunch up your shoulders or lean over to type.

Never hold the telephone between your head and shoulder. Use your hands, a headset model, or a speakerphone.

Keep your upper back and neck straight and your head positioned directly over your neck.

Use armrests to support your forearms.

Slide your buttocks far back in your chair.

Set your chair height so you can keep both feet flat on the ground.

When you sit in a chair to work, ensure that your back is flat against the seat, and your feet are on the floor or propped up on a footrest. Your knees should be slightly below the level of your hips, and your elbows should be bent at a 90° angle. The top of your computer screen should be at eye level.

▶ Proper lifting technique

Try to use your legs as much as possible when lifting something heavy. Also avoid reaching up to grab a weighty object. Instead, get a step stool or platform to put yourself level with the object. This will allow you to use other muscles, in addition to your shoulders, to bear the item's weight.

Ask your employer if the company would purchase an adjustable chair for you. If they won't buy you a chair, invest in one yourself. Adjust the height so that your knees are slightly below your hips with your feet planted firmly on the floor or on a footrest. Your wrists should slope slightly downward, and your elbows should form a 90° angle. Place your back flat against the chair cushion until it is supported. Using a lumbar support pillow will encourage you to sit up straight. When you do sit straight, your eyes should be exactly level with the top of your computer monitor. Keep your mouse close to you so that you don't have to reach, which can overstress your rotator cuff.

When looking at your smartphone or tablet, hold it up so that it is at eye level. Use your other arm to prop up the holding arm if that is more comfortable.

No matter how ergonomic your desk is, don't sit at it for hours at a time. Get up about once every 30 minutes. Walk around and stretch your neck and shoulders to reduce the load and tension on them. You can also use an adjustable desk that lets you alternate between sitting and standing positions. Standing periodically throughout the day will engage the muscles that support your back and shoulders, while also helping to combat some of the ailments associated with a sedentary lifestyle.

If you have transitioned to a standing desk, as an increasing number of American workers have, your new position brings ergonomic challenges of its own. Stand on a padded mat and wear comfortable shoes to protect your feet. Don't lock your knees, but keep them slightly bent. Periodically raise one leg by putting your foot on a small stool or footrest to ease pressure on your back. Position your keyboard so that you can type without bending your wrists, and place your monitor so that the top sits just below your eye level, so that you can stand straight rather than having to lean over. Keep your arms at a 90° angle as you work. Standing isn't the same as moving. Continue to take regular breaks and walk around the office, just as you would if you were sitting all day.

If you can't remember to check your posture regularly on your own, set an alarm on your phone or watch a few times a day to remind you.

Three short exercises to improve shoulder position

A few simple exercises can accustom your body to remaining in the correct posture. Following are brief descriptions. Try practicing these several times during the day. The complete set will take only a few minutes.

Shoulder rolls. Standing up straight with your arms down by your sides, roll your shoulders up, forward, down, and back. Repeat 10 to 15 times. Then reverse the move, rolling your shoulders up, back, down, and forward.

Wall stand. To put your shoulders into the correct alignment, stand with your back against a wall. Make sure that your hips, upper back, and head are all pressed firmly to the wall. Move your shoulder blades down and back until they lightly pinch. Return to the starting position. Repeat 10 to 15 times.

Relaxation series. Many of us naturally hold a lot of tension in our upper back, neck, and shoulders. To release it, try this exercise. Lift your chin slightly and roll your shoulders back until they pinch slightly together. Slowly nod your head "yes" five times, and then shake your head "no" five times. Shrug your shoulders toward your ears and then return to the starting position.

You can find a complete shoulder workout to strengthen shoulders in the Special Section, beginning on page 33. Also see "Proper lifting technique," above left. ▼

The editors would like to thank Casey Vandale, P.T., D.P.T., Senior Physical Therapist, Outpatient Service, Massachusetts General Hospital, and Catherine Schroeder, P.T., D.P.T., O.C.S., Physical Therapist, Massachusetts General Hospital, for their guidance on posture, physical therapy, and rehabilitation.

Diagnosing shoulder pain

Minor shoulder pain that is related to overexertion or a small injury often can be easily managed on your own at home. Because the shoulder is not a weight-bearing joint, you may be able to tough out any discomfort longer than you would be able to with a knee or hip injury. However, more severe pain and limited motion in the shoulder can disrupt your life enough to warrant a call to your doctor. And an injury that might have fractured a bone or torn soft tissue requires urgent care.

Which doctor should you see?

A visit to your primary care doctor is a good first step, unless you think you have a fracture, tear, or another more severe injury. In that case, visit an urgent care center or emergency room for immediate treatment.

Most primary care doctors can assess shoulder symptoms, take x-rays, and determine whether the problem can be treated with conservative measures such as rest and over-the-counter pain relievers, or if it requires further evaluation from an orthopedic specialist.

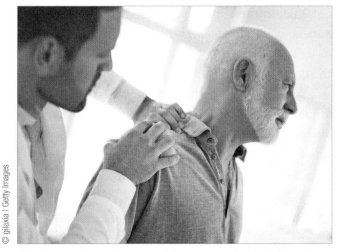

If you're wondering what type of doctor to see for shoulder pain, your primary care physician is a good person to start with. He or she can make an initial evaluation and refer you to a speciaist, if needed.

An orthopedic specialist diagnoses and treats disorders of the bones, joints, ligaments, nerves, and tendons—including sports injuries, other types of trauma, and arthritis. Some orthopedic doctors treat disorders throughout the body, such as the hips, knees, spine, and shoulders. Others focus on the shoulders or another specific area of the body.

Even though these specialists are often referred to as orthopedic surgeons, they won't perform surgery unless it is absolutely necessary to treat your condition or relieve your pain. Instead, they will start with more conservative treatments such as rest, activity modification, physical therapy, and over-the-counter medications.

Many orthopedic offices are busy, which means you might have to wait a few weeks or months to get an appointment with the doctor. However, most practices should have physician's assistants and nurse practitioners who can provide a diagnosis and a recommendation for treatment until you can get an appointment with the orthopedist.

Medical history and exam

Any visit to a doctor should start with a thorough medical history and physical exam. First, the doctor will ask about symptoms such as pain, stiffness, swelling, difficulty with movement, or shoulder joint instability (see "Questions the doctor will ask about your symptoms," page 28). The doctor will also inquire about any injuries you might have sustained to the affected shoulder from sports, work, or accidents.

The doctor will suspect a particular problem based on your symptoms and history. For example, chronic pain and a loss of range of motion from repeated throwing might suggest a frozen shoulder or rotator cuff injury, while a fall with significant pain could indicate a shoulder dislocation or fracture. The doctor should also ask about your other symptoms, such as

© gilaxia | Getty Images

neck or arm pain (which may be a sign of a cervical spine disorder) or chest pain (which could indicate a heart problem).

Next, you'll undergo a physical exam. The doctor will look at your shoulder, checking for signs like swelling, unevenness between the two shoulders, and instability. He or she will feel around your shoulder joints to see if you have any pain or tenderness. You will likely be asked to move the affected shoulder, or the doctor will move your shoulder into one or more positions to compare the range of motion between the affected and unaffected shoulder.

These are several of the tests that doctors use to diagnose shoulder pain:

Abduction. Raise your arm as high as you can out to the side without feeling pain. *Purpose:* To diagnose AC joint problems.

External rotation. Raise your arms to shoulder height in front of your body. Then bend your elbows to a 90° angle, with your palms facing in. Move your arms out to your side, keeping the upper arm parallel to the floor. *Purpose:* To diagnose problems with the teres minor or infraspinatus muscle.

Internal rotation. Raise your arms to shoulder height in front of your body. Then bend your elbows to a 90° angle, with your palms facing in. Move your arms inward, so that the palms and forearms touch.

Questions the doctor will ask about your symptoms

When you're planning to see your primary care doctor or an orthopedic specialist, jot down the answers to the following questions about your shoulder pain, so you'll be prepared to answer them for your doctor:

- When did the pain start?
- Did it start suddenly, or did it develop slowly?
- What were you doing when the pain started?
- Where in the shoulder does it hurt?
- Does the pain radiate to your neck, arms, or elsewhere?
- What is the nature of the pain? Sharp, dull, achy, etc.?
- What other symptoms do you have? Weakness, stiffness, crackling sounds, swelling, bruising, etc.?
- What makes the pain better or worse?

Purpose: To diagnose problems with the subscapularis muscle.

Scarf test. With the affected arm, reach over to touch the opposite shoulder. *Purpose:* To diagnose problems with the AC joint.

Apley scratch test. Reach behind your head and touch the opposite shoulder blade. *Purpose:* To diagnose range-of-motion problems in the shoulder.

Empty can test. Hold your arms out to the side at about 45° with your thumbs pointing downward. Try to raise your arms while the doctor presses down on them. *Purpose:* To diagnose tears to the supraspinatus tendon or muscle.

Lift-off test. Place the affected arm behind your back with the palm facing outward. Push out against the doctor's hand. *Purpose:* To diagnose subscapularis tears or tendinitis.

Blood tests

It might seem strange to have your doctor request a blood sample when your shoulder hurts, but laboratory tests can help diagnose certain conditions.

If rheumatoid arthritis is a possible cause of your pain, a blood test can check for high levels of antinuclear antibodies—a type of immune system protein that mistakenly attacks your own body when you have an autoimmune disease.

An erythrocyte sedimentation rate (ESR) test measures the speed at which erythrocytes (red blood cells) fall to the bottom of a test tube. A faster-than-normal ESR indicates that you have inflammation in your body from a condition such as polymyalgia rheumatica.

If your shoulder pain is part of a group of symptoms that suggests a problem with your heart, gallbladder, or another organ, blood tests can help identify the cause.

Imaging tests

Sometimes your doctor needs a way to see inside your shoulder in order to determine what is causing your pain. The following imaging tests are commonly used to diagnose shoulder problems.

X-rays. An x-ray uses a small dose of ionizing radiation to create images of the bones in your shoulder joint. The density of bone blocks the radiation, making it appear white on the image. Soft tissues like muscle and fat allow more x-rays to pass through, so they appear gray.

Your doctor might recommend an x-ray if you have fallen or had an incident that might have resulted in a fracture, separation, or another bone injury. If your symptoms have lasted for more than four weeks, an x-ray can be a helpful tool for diagnosing arthritis. Narrowing of the joint space and bony overgrowths—both of which are signs of arthritis—will show up on the x-ray image.

To provide your doctor with a clearer image of your joint, a contrast dye may be injected into your shoulder before the x-ray is taken. This test is called arthrography.

Magnetic resonance imaging (MRI). MRI uses powerful magnets, radio waves, and a computer to create images of the bones, tendons, blood vessels, and other structures inside your shoulder. This test is helpful for diagnosing rotator cuff tears, degenerative diseases like arthritis, and sometimes fractures. It can also help your doctor plan out surgery or evaluate the effectiveness of a procedure you have already undergone. During this test, you'll lie on your back on a table, which will slide head-first into the tunnel-like machine. The machine makes loud banging and humming noises during the scan. You'll get earplugs to help mask the

Table 1: Treatments for shoulder pain

Below are some of the common treatments recommended for each cause of shoulder pain. The specific treatment your doctor suggests will be based on factors such as the severity of the problem, how it affects your life, and your personal preferences. All of the treatments mentioned in this table are discussed in more detail in the following chapters.

SHOULDER CONDITION	POSSIBLE TREATMENTS
Arthritis	*Conservative:* Rest, activity modification, physical therapy, exercise, and ice or moist heat *Medication:* Nonsteroidal anti-inflammatory drugs (NSAIDs); disease-modifying drugs such as methotrexate (Trexall) if you have rheumatoid arthritis *Surgery:* AC joint resection, distal clavicle resection (Mumford procedure), shoulder resurfacing, shoulder replacement
Biceps tendon tear	*Conservative:* Ice, rest, physical therapy *Medication:* NSAIDs *Surgery:* Biceps tenodesis
Bursitis	*Conservative:* Rest, activity modification, physical therapy, exercise *Medication:* NSAIDs, corticosteroid injection *Surgery:* Arthroscopy
Dislocation	Closed reduction will be done to put the ball back into the socket. Then the shoulder may be immobilized in a sling. After the sling is removed, you will need rehabilitation to restore movement to the shoulder. *Conservative:* Rest, ice, physical therapy, bracing *Medication:* Over-the-counter or prescription pain relievers *Surgery:* Labrum repair, Bankart repair, SLAP repair
Fracture	*Conservative:* Immobilization with a sling, ice *Medication:* Over-the-counter or prescription pain relievers *Surgery:* ORIF fracture repair with plates, screws, or pins
Frozen shoulder	*Conservative:* Physical therapy *Medication:* NSAIDs, corticosteroid injection *Surgery:* Arthroscopic capsular release
Impingement	*Conservative:* Ice, physical therapy *Medication:* NSAIDs *Surgery:* Shoulder decompression
Rotator cuff injury	*Conservative:* Rest, activity modification, physical therapy, exercise *Medication:* NSAIDs, corticosteroid injection *Surgery:* Arthroscopic or open rotator cuff repair
Separated shoulder	*Conservative:* Rest, ice, sling, physical therapy *Medication:* NSAIDs *Surgery:* AC joint separation repair
Tendinitis	*Conservative:* Rest, ice, physical therapy *Medication:* NSAIDs, corticosteroid injection *Surgery:* Arthroscopy, open surgery

sound or perhaps noise-canceling earphones though which you can hear your choice of music. The entire scan should take about 30 minutes.

In a variation of MRI known as magnetic resonance arthrography, a contrast dye is injected into the joint before the scan. This imaging test provides your doctor with a clearer view of your shoulder, which can be helpful for detecting partial rotator cuff tears.

Computed tomography (CT) scan. A CT scan uses x-rays and computer technology to create cross-sectional images (sometimes called slices) of your shoulder. You lie on a table, while the machine moves in a circle around your body to get multiple views of your shoulder from different angles. A CT scan can reveal in greater detail than an x-ray the bones and soft tissues of your shoulder. It can be helpful for diagnosing fractures that are not visible on an x-ray, as well as arthritis and soft tissue injuries.

Ultrasound. Ultrasound uses sound waves, which bounce back from the structures inside your body to produce an image on a computer screen. In the shoulder, ultrasound is useful for evaluating soft tissue injuries such as rotator cuff tears and biceps tendon tears. During this test, the technician glides a device called a transducer over the parts of your shoulder that are being visualized. You may be asked to move your arm into various positions so the technician can capture images from different angles. The test takes 15 to 30 minutes in total. Afterward, a radiologist will read the images and send a report to the doctor who requested the test. Ultrasound has advantages over other tests in that it is less expensive than MRI and it does not expose your body to radiation as an x-ray or CT scan does.

Electrical studies

If you are experiencing symptoms like numbness, tingling, and weakness, your doctor might also do electrodiagnostic testing to determine whether you have a nerve or muscle disorder. These tests evaluate the speed of electrical signals to and from your brain and muscles. You will typically be referred to either a neurologist or a physiatrist (a physical medicine and rehabilitation specialist) for these tests.

Electromyography measures the electrical activity in your muscles when they are at rest or contracted. This test is done in two parts. During the first part, which is called a nerve conduction study, the technician stimulates the nerves with small electric shocks. The second part—the needle exam—involves inserting a tiny electrode-containing needle into the muscle to read the signals coming from the muscle. You may be asked to lift your arm or perform other actions that make the muscles contract. A healthy, normal muscle should not produce signals while at rest. With modern electromyography studies, needles aren't used as often as they were in the past.

Nerve conduction studies measure the speed at which electrical signals travel down nerve pathways, as well as the strength of those signals. The doctor stimulates your nerve with a mild electrical impulse, and electrode patches placed on your skin record how quickly the signal travels. Damage to a nerve will slow and weaken the nerve signal. Nerve conduction studies can help your doctor find the damaged nerve.

Creating your treatment plan

Once your doctor has discovered the cause of your pain and other symptoms, you will work together to develop a personalized treatment plan (see Table 1, page 29). The goal is to use the least invasive treatment possible to relieve your pain and improve your mobility.

Often, you will start with conservative measures such as rest, activity modification, physical therapy, and over-the-counter pain relievers. If that is not enough, the next step is to graduate to prescription pain relievers, anti-inflammatory drugs, or corticosteroid injections. If none of these strategies relieves your pain or improves your movement, you may need to consider surgery. Make sure you are aware of all your treatment options, as well as the risks involved, before deciding to undergo a procedure. ◗

Conservative (nonsurgical) treatments

When it comes to treating shoulder pain, less is more. Provided your shoulder pain wasn't caused by severe arthritis or an injury like a serious rotator cuff tear or a fracture with displaced bones, you don't have to rush into surgery. In fact, conservative measures such as activity modification, rest, ice or heat, and physical therapy are often the first treatments doctors recommend. Anti-inflammatory pain relievers can also help (see "Drug treatments," page 40). In many cases, these interventions will relieve pain and help you recover movement without the need for more invasive therapies.

Rest and activity modification

One of the easiest treatments for shoulder pain is not a treatment at all. Simply removing the burden from the affected shoulder will give it time to heal and prevent reinjury.

Depending on what condition caused your pain, rest can mean taking a break from any activities that contributed to your injury. Avoid heavy lifting, reaching above shoulder height, and moving into any posi-

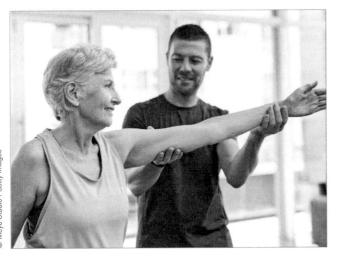

Physical therapy is a cornerstone of shoulder treatment and can even be an alternative to surgery for people with small rotator cuff tears. The goal is to help you regain strength and movement.

tions that worsen your pain. If you work in a job that requires overhead motions or heavy lifting, you might need to take time off or request a change in responsibilities. Athletes may need to stay on the bench until healing is complete.

For some injuries (including fractures), your doctor might recommend keeping the affected shoulder still by putting it in a sling or other shoulder immobilizer. Do not use a sling without your doctor's guidance, however, because too much immobility when you don't need it could slow your recovery and possibly lead to frozen shoulder (see page 21). If you do need a sling, your doctor should show you how to use it correctly. Improperly worn slings can actually increase the pressure on your injured shoulder and further compromise your recovery. You want the sling to support your arm and shoulder without being too tight. Your shoulder, elbow, and wrist should be in a comfortable position, with your elbow bent at a 90° angle.

Ice and heat

Ice and heat are two other easy interventions for relieving shoulder pain, but which one is best? That depends on your injury and when you sustained it.

Immediately after an injury, ice helps to bring down inflammation and numbs pain. For the first 24 to 48 hours after the injury, place an ice pack or cold compress on the affected shoulder for 15 to 20 minutes at a time every three to four hours. You can use something as simple as a package of frozen peas for a makeshift ice pack. Whatever you use, do not place the pack directly on the skin. This can lead to frostbite.

Once the swelling has subsided, switch to heat. A heating pad eases stiff muscles and joints, and it increases blood flow to the area. For arthritis pain, try moist heat—for example, from a warm wet washcloth.

© Moyo Studio | Getty Images

Physical therapy

Physical therapy is a cornerstone of shoulder treatment. The goal of physical therapy is to help you regain strength and movement in the affected shoulder, so that activities such as reaching to pull an item off a shelf or putting on your shirt become easier and less painful.

Physical therapy can be an alternative to surgery for people with small rotator cuff tears and mild to moderate osteoarthritis. Rotator cuff tears will not heal on their own, but physical therapy can help some people improve their biomechanics, restore function, build strength, and reduce pain to the extent that surgery is not necessary. In fact, a study in *The Bone & Joint Journal* found physical therapy to be just as effective as surgery for most people with small tears. Therapy can also speed your recovery after surgery (see "Post-surgery rehabilitation," page 50).

To start, you will need a prescription from your primary care provider or an orthopedic specialist. If your doctor does not suggest physical therapy, ask if it is an option for you. Most insurance plans, including Medicare and Medicaid, will cover the cost for a specific number of sessions.

Ideally, you should see a physical therapist who has specific expertise in treating shoulder injuries.

Your first visit will start with a comprehensive evaluation. The therapist will ask about your medical history, the nature of your injury, and your pain level. Expect to also answer questions about your functional ability—for example, is it difficult for you to put on a shirt or to drive?

Then you will have a full physical assessment. The therapist should check your posture; the position of your head, neck, and cervical spine; and whether your shoulders are in the proper alignment. (Physical therapy exercises can help improve poor posture.) This will be followed by an evaluation of the range of motion in your shoulder joint, both actively (as you move your arm yourself) and passively (as the therapist moves your arm for you). The therapist will check the strength of your rotator cuff and other shoulder muscles, and he or she will look for any loss of function in your elbow and hand.

Although a doctor will usually have examined you first, a physical therapist will also check for potential medical causes of your pain and for neck or back problems that could be the underlying cause of your shoulder pain.

The physical therapy program includes a range of exercises—some that you do with the therapist, others that you do on your own at home—to strengthen and improve mobility in the muscles that support your shoulder joint. You will likely use a combination of light weights, exercise bands, and weight-bearing exercises (such as push-ups or planks), depending on your strength, ability, and stage of recovery. (See the Special Section, "Exercises to prevent and relieve shoulder pain," page 33, for a basic shoulder workout for tendinitis, bursitis, impingement, or osteoarthritis.) Your therapist might also use treatments such as ice, heat, or manual therapy.

Expect to visit your therapist at least once a week for four to six weeks before you start to see any improvements in shoulder pain and function. If your symptoms have not improved in about six weeks, you may need to see an orthopedic specialist to discuss other treatment options. ▼

Exercises to prevent and relieve shoulder pain

Following a minor shoulder injury, or when you live with arthritis, regular exercise can strengthen the muscles that support your shoulder and help prevent future injuries. A home exercise program should incorporate all of the main muscles in your shoulder, including the deltoid, biceps, trapezius, supraspinatus, infraspinatus, and subscapularis muscles (see "The rotator cuff, shoulder muscles, and other structures," page 10). Adding flexibility or stretching exercises will help you regain range of motion in the joint so you can get back to your previous work or activities.

In this chapter you'll find a complete shoulder workout, including warm-ups and stretches in addition to strengthening exercises. This workout is excerpted from *The Joint Pain Relief Workout: Healing Exercises for Your Shoulders, Hips, Knees, and Ankles* by Lauren E. Elson, physical medicine and rehabilitation instructor at Harvard Medical School. (For information on the full report, see "Resources," page 52.)

Note: This workout is specifically for people with shoulder impingement, osteoarthritis, bursitis, or tendinitis. If you have other shoulder conditions or have

recently had surgery, do not try these exercises, but consult a physical therapist for a series of exercises specific to your condition. If you *do* have one of the conditions this workout is designed to treat,

it's still a good idea to show a copy of these exercises to your doctor or a physical therapist and ask whether these are safe for you. And if you feel any pain while doing these exercises, stop immediately and call your doctor for guidance.

Assuming you are cleared for this exercise program, here's how to follow it.

For the first two weeks: Do only the warm-ups and stretches. Practice at least two to three times a week or as often as daily.

Starting at week 3: Begin to perform the full workout two to three times a week. Make sure you leave 48 hours between strength

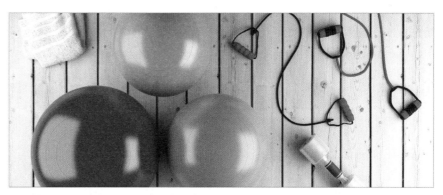

Shoulder exercises do not require a lot of equipment. Light hand weights (1 to 3 pounds) and resistance tubing with a door attachment are all you really need. Stability balls are optional.

© Eoneren | Getty Images

exercise sessions to allow muscles time to recover. Warm-ups and stretches can be done daily to further enhance flexibility.

Equipment: 1- to 3-pound hand weights, resistance tubing with door attachment, hand towel, stability ball (optional). Note that resistance tubing comes with padded handles on the ends, and in different colors to designate varying amounts of resistance, from very light to very heavy. For this workout, choose light to medium resistance. Also look for a brand with a door attachment, which allows you to anchor the tubing in place when doing certain exercises, such as "Standing row" (page 37).

If you are not used to reading exercise instructions, some of the terminology may be unfamiliar to you. Here's what the terms mean:

Starting position. This describes how to position your body before starting the exercise.

Movement. Here you'll find out how to perform the exercise correctly.

Repetitions (reps). Each time you complete the full movement, that's a rep. It's fine if you can't do all the reps at first. Focus on quality—good form comes first—rather than quantity. Gradually increase reps as you improve.

Sets. One set is a specific number of repetitions. In our workouts, 10 reps typically add up to a single set.

Intensity. Intensity measures how hard you're working during an exercise.

Tempo. This provides the pace for the key movements in an exercise. Here's how the 3-1-3 tempo works in "Wall push-up with stability ball" (page 35): Slowly count to three while bending your elbows to lower your upper body toward the wall. Pause for one second. Then count to three again as you return to the starting position.

Hold. Hold tells you the number of seconds to maintain a pose during a stretch.

Rest. Resting gives your muscles a chance to recharge, which helps you maintain good form.

1. Warming up: Shoulder circles

Reps: 20 per arm (10 in each direction)   **Tempo:** Slow and controlled

Sets: 1   **Rest:** No rest needed

Intensity: Light

Starting position: Stand up straight with your feet hip-width apart. Hold a 1- to 3-pound weight in your right hand with one end of the weight hanging down toward the floor.

Movement: Bend your knees a bit and slightly hinge forward from the hip so that you're holding the weight between your legs. You can rest your left hand on your left thigh for support. Make 10 clockwise circles with your right arm as if stirring a pot. Pause, then reverse direction for 10 circles. Move the weight to your left hand and repeat the sequence. This completes one set.

Tips and techniques:

• Hinge from the hips without bending or arching your back.

• Keep your shoulder blades down and back.

• Allow the weight to hang as a dead weight.

Make it easier: Perform the exercise while seated, or try it standing with no weight.

Make it harder: Make larger circles.

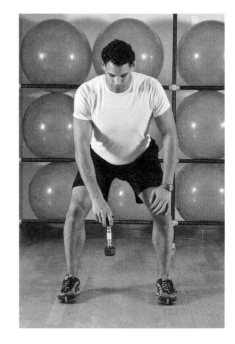

2. Warming up: Shoulder pendulums

Reps: 10 per side

Sets: 1

Intensity: Light

Tempo: Slow and controlled

Rest: No rest needed

Starting position: Stand up straight with your feet together. Hold a 1- to 3-pound weight in your right hand with your arm at your side and one end of the weight hanging down toward the floor.

Movement: Extend your right leg behind you and press the right heel toward the floor, bending your left knee slightly and hinging forward at your hips. Place your left hand on your left thigh for support. Slowly rock your body forward and back, causing the weight to swing gently like a pendulum. Each forward-and-back swing is one rep. Finish all reps, then switch leg position and repeat with the weight in your left hand. This completes one set.

Tips and techniques:

- Maintain a neutral spine, and keep your shoulders down and back, not hunched up by your ears.
- Let the rocking power the movement of the weight instead of using your shoulder to swing the weight.

- As you rock forward, let your back heel lift off the floor. As you rock backward, let the toes of your front leg lift off the floor as your back heel comes down.

Make it easier: Perform the exercise while seated, or try it standing with no weight.

Make it harder: Make a larger arc as you swing the weight like a pendulum.

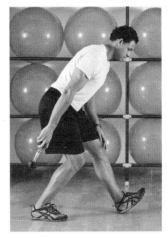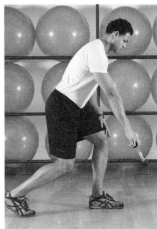

3. Strengthening: Wall push-up with stability ball

Reps: 10

Sets: 1–3

Intensity: Moderate to hard

Tempo: 3-1-3

Rest: 30–90 seconds between sets

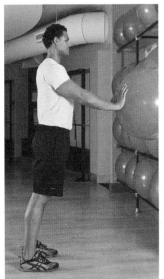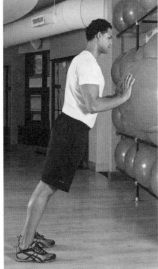

Starting position: Facing a wall, stand up straight and position a stability ball against the wall at chest height. (If you do not have a stability ball, you can do this exercise against the wall.) Extend your arms at chest height with your palms against the ball, fingertips pointing toward the ceiling.

Movement: Slowly bend your elbows to lower your upper body toward the ball, keeping a straight line from head to heel. Pause, then slowly push away from the ball to return to the starting position. This is one rep.

Tips and techniques:

- Keep your fingertips no higher than shoulder level.
- Keep your elbows close to your sides as you bend them.
- Throughout the movement, maintain neutral alignment from head to toe, with your shoulders down and back.

Make it easier: Try the wall push-up without the stability ball.

Make it harder: After you lower your body toward the ball, hold the position for a count of eight. Then slowly push away from the ball to return to the starting position.

4. Strengthening: Standing internal and external rotation

Reps: 10 of each step per side

Sets: 1–3

Intensity: Moderate

Tempo: 3-1-3

Rest: 30–90 seconds between sets

Starting position: Anchor the resistance tubing to a door at waist level. Stand with the door on your right side and your feet hip-width apart. Grasp one handle of the tubing in your right hand with your thumb pointed at the ceiling and your elbow firmly pinning a rolled-up hand towel at your side. Adjust where you are standing so the band is taut.

Movement: This is a two-step exercise.

Step 1: Keep your wrist aligned with your arm (don't bend it) as you slowly pull the band in toward your belly button like a door closing. Pause, then slowly return to the starting position. Finish all reps.

Step 2: Switch hands so that you are grasping the handle with your left hand across your waist, knuckles near your belly button, and your left elbow pinning the hand towel at your left side. (If necessary, adjust the tension on the resistance tubing by moving a bit closer to or farther away from the door.) Keep your wrist straight as you slowly pull the tubing outward like a door opening. Pause, then slowly return to the starting position. Finish all reps. Turn your body so the door is on your left side and repeat both steps. This completes one set.

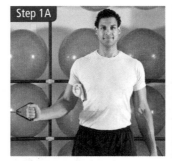

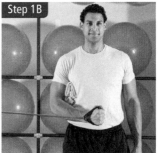

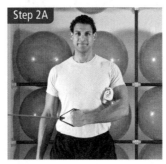

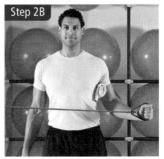

Tips and techniques:

• Maintain neutral posture, with your shoulders down and back.

• Note that the motion should come from the shoulder joint only. Hips should remain stationary at all times.

• Maintain a firm, neutral wrist; don't bend your wrist.

Make it easier: Use lighter resistance tubing.

Make it harder: Use heavier resistance tubing.

5. Strengthening: Standing V-raise

Reps: 10

Sets: 1–3

Intensity: Moderate

Tempo: 3-1-3

Rest: 30–90 seconds between sets

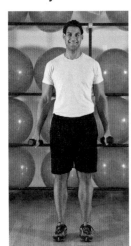

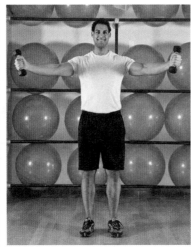

Starting position: Stand up straight holding a 1- to 3-pound weight in each hand with your arms at your sides, thumbs facing forward. Position your feet hip-width apart.

Movement: Squeeze your shoulder blades together while you slowly lift your arms, creating a V as you raise the weights to shoulder height. Pause, then slowly return to the starting position. This is one rep.

Tips and techniques:

• Keep your wrists aligned with your arms, maintaining a straight line from your elbow to your knuckles.

• Maintain neutral posture, with your shoulders down and back. Don't pull your shoulders up toward your ears as you lift.

• Keep your elbows soft (not locked) throughout the movement.

Make it easier: Use a lighter weight.

Make it harder: Use a heavier weight.

6. Strengthening: Standing row

Reps: 10

Sets: 1–3

Intensity: Moderate

Tempo: 3-1-3

Rest: 30–90 seconds between sets

Starting position: Anchor the middle of the resistance tubing to a door at about waist height and grasp a handle in each hand. Stand up straight facing the door with your feet together. Stand far enough away from the door to put tension on the tubing as you hold the handles with your arms extended. Extend your right leg straight back and press the right heel toward the floor, bending both knees slightly.

Movement: Squeeze your shoulder blades together. Slowly bend your arms and pull back. Keep your elbows close to your ribs and pointing behind you. Pause, then slowly return to the starting position. This is one rep.

Tips and techniques:
• Maintain neutral posture, with your shoulders down and back.

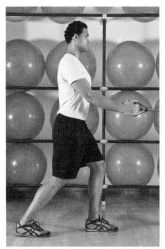
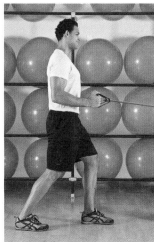

• Keep your wrists straight; don't bend them.
• Contract your abdominal muscles.

Make it easier: Use lighter resistance tubing.

Make it harder: Use heavier resistance tubing.

7. Strengthening: Biceps curl

Reps: 10

Sets: 1–3

Intensity: Light to moderate

Tempo: 3-1-3

Rest: 30–90 seconds between sets

Starting position: Stand up straight with your feet hip-width apart, holding 1- to 3-pound weights at your side with your palms facing forward.

Movement: Slowly bend your elbows to lift the weights up in front of your shoulders. Exhale as you lift. Pause. Slowly lower them to the starting position. This is one rep.

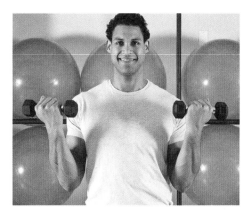

Tips and techniques:
• Keep your shoulders still, down, and back.
• Keep your wrists straight; don't bend them as you lift.
• Keep your upper arms stationary and your elbows at your sides throughout the movement.

Make it easier: Use lighter weights.

Make it harder: Use heavier weights.

8. Strengthening: Diagonals

Reps: 10 of each step per side

Tempo: 3-1-3

Sets: 1–3

Rest: 30–90 seconds between sets

Intensity: Moderate

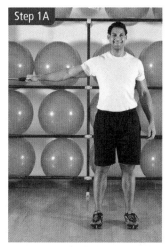
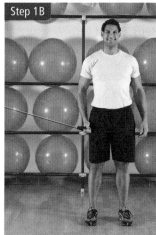

Step 1A · Step 1B

Starting position: Anchor the resistance tubing to a door at chest level. Stand with your right side to the door. Position your legs hip-width apart, chest up, and shoulders down and back. Grasp the handle of the tubing horizontally in your right hand with your arm held out straight just below shoulder height, palm down. Keep tension on the tubing throughout the exercise.

Movement: This is a two-step exercise.

Step 1: Keeping your wrist firm and arm straight, slowly pull your right arm down toward your right hip. Pause, then slowly return to the starting position. Finish all reps, then stand with your left side to the door and repeat, grasping the handle in your left hand.

Step 2: Anchor the resistance tubing to the floor by stepping on it with your left foot. Hold the handle with your right hand near your left hip, palm facing you. Adjust the length of the tubing so it is taut. Keeping your wrist firm and arm straight, slowly lift your right hand up on a diagonal to shoulder height, palm facing forward. Pause, then slowly bring your right hand back to your left hip. Finish all reps with the right arm before anchoring the tubing under your right foot and repeating with your left arm. This completes one set.

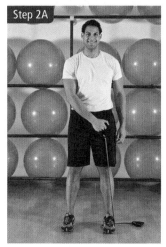
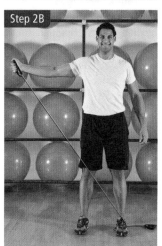

Step 2A · Step 2B

Tips and techniques:

• You may need to use lighter resistance tubing on this exercise to complete the movement with good form and ease.

• Keep your wrist straight; don't bend it as you pull.

• Maintain neutral posture, with your shoulders down and back.

Make it easier: Use lighter resistance tubing.

Make it harder: Use heavier resistance tubing.

9. Stretching: Shoulder stretch

Reps: 3–4 per side

Sets: 1

Intensity: Light

Hold: 10–30 seconds

Rest: No rest needed

Starting position: Stand with your feet hip-width apart. Put your left hand on your right shoulder. Cup your left elbow with your right hand.

Movement: Roll your shoulders down and back as you gently pull your left elbow across your chest. Hold. Return to the starting position. Finish all reps, then repeat on the other side. This completes one set.

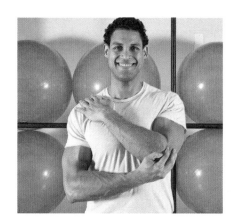

Tips and techniques:

• Stretch to the point of mild tension, not pain.

• Keep your shoulders down and back.

• Don't twist as you stretch.

Make it easier: Stretch only as far as is comfortable.

Make it harder: Repeat the stretch several times during the day.

10. Stretching: Wall climb

Reps: 3–4 of each step per side

Sets: 1

Intensity: Light to moderate

Hold: 10–30 seconds

Rest: No rest needed

Starting position: Stand up straight facing a wall.

Movement: This is a two-part exercise.

Step 1: Extend your right arm with your elbow soft (not locked) and place your hand on the wall at shoulder height. Slowly walk your fingers upward, stepping in toward the wall as your hand climbs higher. Stop when you feel mild tension in your shoulder. Hold. Slowly walk your fingers back down the wall and return to the starting position. Finish all reps. Switch arms and repeat.

Step 2: Turn so that your left side faces the wall. Extend your left arm with your elbow soft (not locked) and place your hand on the wall at shoulder height. Slowly walk your fingers upward, stepping in toward the wall as your hand climbs higher. Stop when you feel mild tension in your shoulder. Hold. Slowly walk your fingers back down the wall and return to the starting position. Finish all reps. Switch arms and repeat. This completes one set.

Tips and techniques:
- Stretch to the point of mild tension, not pain.
- Progress slowly toward the goal of bringing your body right next to the wall.
- Breathe comfortably.

Make it easier: Place your hand on the wall below shoulder height and go only as high as is comfortable.

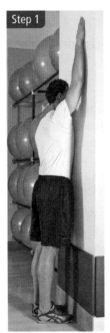 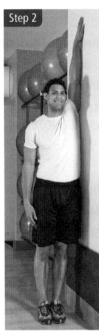

Make it harder: Repeat the stretch several times throughout the day.

11. Stretching: Shoulder stretch with internal rotation

Reps: 3–4 per side

Sets: 1

Intensity: Moderate

Hold: 10–30 seconds

Rest: No rest needed

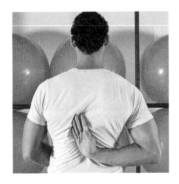

Starting position: Stand up straight with your feet hip-width apart and your hands by your sides.

Movement: Place the back of your right hand against the small of your back at your waist. Your fingers should be pointing up. Slowly slide your right hand farther up your back as high as you can. Hold. Finish all reps, then repeat with your left hand. This completes one set.

Tips and techniques:
- Stretch to the point of mild tension, not pain.
- Maintain neutral posture, with your shoulders down and back.
- Breathe comfortably.

Make it easier: Make your movement smaller.

Make it harder: Repeat the stretch several times during the day.

12. Stretching: Chest stretch

Reps: 3–4 per side

Sets: 1

Intensity: Light to moderate

Hold: 10–30 seconds

Rest: No rest needed

Starting position: Stand alongside a doorway or wall. Extend your right arm and put your right hand on the edge of the door frame slightly below shoulder level, palm facing forward and touching the door frame. Keep your shoulders down and back.

Movement: Slowly turn your body to the left, away from the door frame, until you feel the stretch in your chest and shoulder. Hold. Return to the starting position. Finish all reps, then repeat on the opposite side. This completes one set.

Tips and techniques:
- Keep your shoulders back and down.
- Stretch to the point of mild tension, not pain.
- Breathe comfortably.

Make it easier: Make your movement smaller.

Make it harder: Repeat the stretch several times during the day. ◆

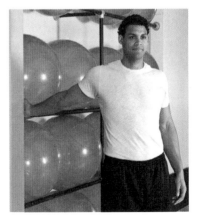

Drug treatments

Pain is a hallmark of shoulder dysfunction and injury. Depending on the cause of your injury, the discomfort can be severe enough to interrupt your daily routine and keep you awake at night. Both over-the-counter and prescription pain relievers can be very effective tools for alleviating shoulder-related pain, especially when you use them in conjunction with nondrug treatments, such as physical therapy, as outlined earlier in this report.

More experimental therapies, such as platelet-rich plasma injections and stem cell treatments, are also available. However, the evidence on these treatments is mixed (see "Stem cell treatments: Do they work?" below).

Anti-inflammatories and pain relievers

Nonsteroidal anti-inflammatory drugs (NSAIDs) are among the most commonly used pain relievers in the world. Most people are familiar with the over-the-counter NSAID varieties—aspirin, ibuprofen (Advil, Motrin), and naproxen (Aleve). Prescription-strength NSAIDs are also available. Among them are diclofenac (Cataflam, Voltaren), etodolac (Lodine), indomethacin (Indocin, Tivorbex), meloxicam (Mobic), nabumetone (Relafen), naproxen (Anaprox, Naprosyn), and piroxicam (Feldene).

This class of drug is particularly useful for treating inflammatory diseases such as arthritis because it serves double duty, both relieving pain and bringing down inflammation. These drugs are also helpful for other causes of shoulder pain, including tendinitis and bursitis.

NSAIDs block the action of two enzymes: cyclooxygenase 1 and 2 (COX-1 and COX-2), which produce chemicals called prostaglandins. COX-2 enzymes produce prostaglandins that promote inflammation and pain throughout the body. Blocking them therefore reduces pain. However, stomach irritation is a frequent side effect (see "NSAID side effects," page 41). That's

---

Stem cell treatments: Do they work?

If you do an online search for "stem cell treatments," you will likely bring up a list of websites with futuristic names, offering the promise of revolutionary healing methods. These companies claim they can use your own stem cells to heal injuries like rotator cuff tears or arthritic joint degeneration, without the need for surgery and the lengthy rehabilitation process that follows. Yet the stem cell treatments currently available are not worth their high price tag, which can run into the thousands of dollars for each injection—and typically aren't covered by insurance. What's more, they could be risky.

The promise of stem cells lies in their versatility. These fledgling cells have the potential to differentiate into a variety of cell types, including muscle and cartilage. That makes them a useful part of the body's repair system, regenerating tissues that have been damaged by injury.

A number of clinical trials are investigating the feasibility of using stem cells to treat injuries to the shoulder and other joints. Results so far have been promising. However, the treatments that are currently being marketed to consumers don't use pure stem cells, because they are so challenging to collect. Typically, the stem cells are harvested from a person's bone marrow and bloodstream and then put through a centrifuge to separate out red blood cells, serum, and other components until only

cells with a nucleus remain. In reality, only one out of several thousand cells in a sample will be a stem cell. Most of the material that is ultimately injected into patients' shoulders is therefore useless.

What's more, many of the companies that aggressively market online do not use rigorous preparation methods. Improperly prepared stem cells could potentially cause a dangerous infection or an immune system reaction.

If you are interested in investigating stem cell therapies for a shoulder injury, seek out credible institutions, such as universities that are conducting medical research. Stay away from clinics that you find online—especially ones making claims that sound too good to be true.

---

because COX-1 enzymes produce prostaglandins that exert a protective effect, increasing the production of mucus in the stomach lining and reducing the release of stomach acids. Blocking COX-1 hampers these effects.

There are several options for dealing with potential stomach upset. The prescription NSAID celecoxib (Celebrex) is a selective COX-2 inhibitor, meaning that it primarily targets the COX-2 enzyme without hampering protective COX-1.

Another way to reduce NSAID stomach irritation is to take a proton-pump inhibitor, such as omeprazole (Prilosec), once a day along with your NSAID. Proton-pump inhibitors are drugs designed to treat gastroesophageal reflux by reducing stomach acid. The prescription pain reliever Vimovo is a combination of prescription-strength naproxen and the proton-pump inhibitor esomeprazole (sold on its own as Nexium), but it's just as easy (and cheaper) to take an over-the-counter proton-pump inhibitor with your NSAID.

Another option is acetaminophen (Tylenol), which relieves pain but does not address inflammation and is therefore not an NSAID. Just be careful to stick to the recommended dose (no more than 4,000 milligrams daily, or less for some people). In larger amounts, Tylenol can damage the liver.

Whichever pain reliever you choose, make sure your doctor is aware that you are taking it. Use the lowest possible dose for the shortest period of time needed to manage your shoulder pain.

Narcotic or opioid pain relievers are another pain relief option, but only on a short-term basis immediately after surgery. For chronic pain, they are not recommended, because they come with a host of side effects such as constipation, nausea, and drowsiness, not to mention a high potential for addiction and abuse. Research finds that physical therapy is a better early treatment for most shoulder pain. According to a 2018 study in *JAMA Network Open*,

starting physical therapy shortly after being diagnosed with shoulder pain can help reduce the need for these potentially harmful and addictive drugs.

Corticosteroid injections

Corticosteroids are drugs that mimic the hormone cortisol, which your body makes in response to stress. When injected, these drugs work by dampening the immune response, thereby bringing down inflammation and its resulting pain. By reducing inflammation, the shots also improve range of motion, making it easier to engage in physical therapy or exercise. (Although they are often referred to as "steroids," these drugs aren't the same as the anabolic steroids weight lifters take to boost muscle mass.)

Corticosteroids are injected directly into the injured shoulder, usually in combination with a local

NSAID side effects

Nonsteroidal anti-inflammatory drugs (NSAIDs) are a very effective tool for managing minor arthritis pain or shoulder discomfort from other causes. However, these drugs come with side effects that can make them dangerous when used in larger amounts than recommended or in people with certain medical conditions. These risks increase with higher doses and longer use. Note that it's possible to overdose inadvertently if you're taking more than one product containing an NSAID. Side effects include the following:

Stomach upset and bleeding. Losing the COX-1 enzyme's protective effect on the stomach lining can lead to side effects like abdominal pain, nausea, vomiting, heartburn, gas, diarrhea, ulcers, and bleeding. The risks are higher in people over age 65, those who have a history of stomach ulcers, and those who also take blood thinners or corticosteroids. Celecoxib (Celebrex) is less likely to cause stomach-related side effects.

Heart problems. Back in 2005, the FDA issued a label warning that NSAIDs increase the risks for heart attacks and strokes. In 2015, the agency strengthened this warning, cautioning consumers that heart risks increase as quickly as the first few weeks after people start using these drugs regularly, and they continue to increase with a longer duration of use and at higher doses. The risk is greatest among people with existing heart disease, although even those with a previously healthy heart could have a heart attack or stroke while on these pain relievers. Heart failure is another potential concern with these drugs. Be cautious about using NSAIDs if you have heart disease or a condition like rheumatoid arthritis or diabetes that increases your risk for heart disease. If you need an NSAID, your doctor might recommend naproxen (Aleve) or celecoxib, because these drugs are safer for people at risk for heart disease.

Liver and kidney damage. NSAIDs can affect both liver and kidney function. Your doctor might choose to monitor the function of these organs by giving you blood tests every one to two months while you take these drugs.

anesthetic to provide some immediate pain relief. Research finds these injections offer small, short-term relief from conditions like rotator cuff injuries. However, they may not be much more effective than NSAIDs, and they do come with some risks, such as infection, nerve damage, bone weakening, skin discoloration around the injection site, and a temporary spike in blood sugar levels.

Steroid shots are given in the doctor's office. Your doctor might use ultrasound to guide the needle to the right spot. Afterward, you could have some redness and irritation around the injection site. Your shoulder pain might flare at first, but it should gradually improve. Rarely, complications like nerve damage and joint infection can occur after steroid injections.

Doctors usually recommend limiting corticosteroid injections to no more than three or four per year. More frequent injections can increase cartilage damage within the joint. If you've had four shots and your pain continues, investigate other pain relief options.

DMARDs for rheumatoid arthritis

Rheumatoid arthritis requires a different approach to treatment than osteoarthritis, because pain and joint destruction stem from an autoimmune attack on the joint, rather than from wear and tear. This requires a treatment that calms the overactive immune system and suppresses inflammation.

Treatment guidelines from the American Academy of Rheumatology recommend a disease-modifying antirheumatic drug (DMARD) such as methotrexate (Trexall) as the first treatment. If that does not work, you can add a type of biologic drug called a TNF inhibitor. These drugs target a substance in your blood called TNF, which contributes to joint inflammation. Oral corticosteroids, such as prednisone, are also used temporarily to control inflammation.

Platelet-rich plasma injection

Platelet-rich plasma (PRP) injection is a relatively new and controversial therapy that is meant to speed healing in a damaged joint. The PRP preparation is made of components drawn from your own blood. Plasma is the liquid portion of blood; it carries red blood cells, white blood cells, and platelets. Platelets help your blood clot: when you have an injury, they rush to the site and stick together to plug up the wound. Platelets also contain growth factors that promote healing. Researchers have been investigating the use of PRP—that is, plasma enriched with extra platelets—for treating musculoskeletal soft tissue injuries, such as rotator cuff tears, frozen shoulder, and impingement.

To treat you with this therapy, the doctor would first draw some of your blood and separate out the platelets from the red and white blood cells. The blood cells are returned to you, while the platelets are run through a machine called a centrifuge to increase their concentration in one portion of the plasma. Boosting the number of platelets also increases the amount of growth factors in the sample. The PRP is then injected into your injured shoulder.

The major question with PRP is whether it works. So far, the research has been promising but inconclusive. It has been difficult for researchers to do any real comparisons because the techniques used to collect and concentrate the platelets have differed, sometimes substantially, from one research group to another. In one study of 20 people with partial rotator cuff tears, patients reported significant improvements in shoulder pain and function eight weeks after the injections, and doctors noted that the injuries had healed well. Other studies have shown no significant effect.

This treatment could offer an alternative for people who can't take corticosteroids, as evidence suggests that it works at least as well as steroid injections. Researchers are also investigating whether PRP might speed healing after shoulder surgery. One randomized controlled study of PRP injections after arthroscopic supraspinatus repair found improvements in strength and patient satisfaction. However, given the relatively small number of people who have been studied so far, more research is needed to confirm whether this treatment can actually make a difference in large numbers of people. Because this therapy is still considered experimental, most insurance companies will not cover the cost, which can run $500 to $1,000 per injection. ▼

Surgery

For most common shoulder problems and injuries, surgery is considered a last resort. Nonsurgical methods like activity modification, physical therapy, exercise, and pain relievers can often alleviate pain and restore movement, enabling you to avoid going under the knife.

However, more severe injuries and problems that cause chronic pain or instability may need to be addressed in a hospital operating room. Here are some of the reasons why your orthopedic surgeon might recommend that you consider having a procedure:

- You have persistent pain or weakness from a torn rotator cuff, and the injury has not improved after three to six months of conservative treatments.
- You have a large rotator cuff tear that could cause permanent muscle deterioration if not fixed.
- Your shoulder pain and loss of movement are interfering with work, sports, or daily activities.
- You have repeatedly dislocated your shoulder and the joint is now unstable.
- You have a severe fracture of the collarbone or upper arm bone that is not likely to heal on its own.
- Your acromioclavicular joint, where the collarbone and shoulder blade meet at the top of your shoulder, has separated.
- Osteoarthritis or rheumatoid arthritis has severely damaged your shoulder joint, causing pain and limiting movement.

It is important to note that the decision to have surgery is not always clear-cut. Your surgeon should let you know whether you meet the general criteria, but your personal preferences and issues related to quality of life will also factor in to your decision. Before deciding to have surgery, do your due diligence to find a qualified, experienced surgeon to ensure the best possible outcome (see "What to look for in a shoulder surgeon," page 44).

Your specific injury and its severity will dictate whether you have a minimally invasive arthroscopic procedure or more extensive open surgery. This chapter explores some of the most commonly performed shoulder surgeries.

Arthroscopy

Arthroscopy is a minimally invasive surgical technique. In the shoulder joint, it's used to repair tendons, ligaments, and cartilage and to remove bone spurs, loose cartilage, or inflamed tissue (see Figure 8, below). The term arthroscopy comes from the Greek words *arthron* ("joint") and *skopein* ("to look"). As the term suggests, the surgeon looks inside your joint with a miniature camera and uses tiny instruments inserted

Figure 8: Shoulder arthroscopy

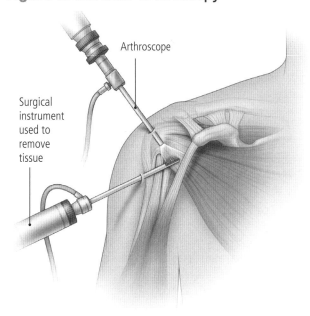

Arthroscope

Surgical instrument used to remove tissue

Shoulder arthroscopy is a minimally invasive procedure used to treat rotator cuff repairs, arthritis, frozen shoulder, torn cartilage, and other damage to the shoulder joint. The surgeon inserts a small camera called an arthroscope into the shoulder. The camera sends an image of the surgical area to a monitor, which the surgeon can view while performing the operation. Tiny instruments inserted into other small incisions in the shoulder are used to make the repair.

through small incisions to perform the surgery.

Arthroscopy has been around since the 1970s, and it is the preferred method for procedures like rotator cuff repair. Performing the operation through smaller incisions typically results in less pain and a faster recovery than does the traditional method, known as open surgery, in which the surgeon makes an incision long enough to view and work on the damaged area directly.

Your doctor might recommend an arthroscopic procedure to

- repair a torn rotator cuff (rotator cuff repair)
- remove or repair a torn labrum—the rim of cartilage lining the shoulder socket (labrum repair, SLAP repair)
- stabilize a joint that has become unstable after repeated dislocations (Bankart repair)
- remove bone spurs or loose cartilage (debridement)
- fix a separated acromioclavicular (AC) joint (AC joint separation repair)

- treat shoulder impingement syndrome (shoulder decompression)
- repair a damaged biceps tendon (biceps tenodesis)
- repair a frozen shoulder (arthroscopic capsular release)
- treat AC joint problems due to arthritis (AC joint resection, distal clavicle excision, or distal clavicle resection)
- treat arthritis damage (shoulder resurfacing).
- Surgeons can also repair a fracture or release an impinged nerve using arthroscopy.

What to expect

Before you have any type of shoulder surgery, your doctor will want to make sure you are healthy enough to undergo the procedure. You may need to have blood tests, x-rays, an electrocardiogram (which measures the heart's electrical activity), and possibly other tests to confirm your fitness for surgery.

What to look for in a shoulder surgeon

Once you have made the decision to have surgery, you need to find a surgeon you trust. Your choice of surgeon has a big impact on your outcome. When looking for a surgeon, start with a referral from your primary care physician or orthopedist. You can also ask friends or family members who have undergone shoulder surgery, but remember that their situation may not mirror your own. Once you have a few names, do some research. Here are a few things to look for:

Board certification in orthopedic surgery. This indicates that the surgeon has training in performing musculoskeletal procedures. You can check your prospective surgeon's certification status on Certification Matters, a website from the American Board of Medical Specialties (www.certificationmatters.org).

Specialization in shoulders. Many shoulder experts have advanced training in shoulders and are members of specialty organizations that require some expertise. Such organizations

include American Shoulder and Elbow Surgeons (www.ases-assn.org), the American Orthopaedic Society for Sports Medicine (www.sportsmed.org), and the Arthroscopy Association of North America (www.aana.org).

A high volume of procedures. Ask how many shoulder surgeries the doctor performs each year. The more, the better. Going to a surgeon who performs these procedures with some regularity (more than 40 procedures per year) and has fellowship training will lower your risk for complications and could lead to a shorter hospital stay and better overall results, research finds.

A clean record. Make sure the doctor has no history of malpractice claims or disciplinary actions. You can check his or her record and get information on the doctor's education, licensing, and certifications on websites such as those provided by Healthgrades (https://www.healthgrades.com) and the Federation of State Medical Boards (www.docinfo.org). Some of these sites include patient satisfaction surveys. Although everyone's

experience with a surgeon is different, a preponderance of negative reviews is a sign that you need to keep looking.

A high-quality hospital. Also evaluate the hospital where you will be having your surgery. You are more likely to have a good outcome at a top-rated hospital. Make sure the hospital is accredited by the Joint Commission (www.qualitycheck.org), a nonprofit organization that focuses on health care quality and safety. You can find hospital ratings through the Leapfrog Group (www.leapfroggroup.org) and *U.S. News & World Report* (https://health.usnews.com/best-hospitals).

A responsive office. The surgeon's office staff should provide consistently high levels of customer service. When you call the office, does a staff member pick up right away, or are you left on hold for many minutes? Are your questions answered in a timely fashion, or can you never seem to reach the doctor? Poor communication and response times before your surgery could foretell trouble afterward.

You will also be asked what medications you take. Some medications—including blood thinners such as heparin, apixaban (Eliquis), rivaroxaban (Xarelto), and warfarin (Coumadin), and pain relievers such as aspirin, ibuprofen (Advil, Motrin), and naproxen (Aleve)—must be stopped a week or so before surgery because they can increase your bleeding risk during the procedure. Your surgeon's staff will give you instructions on when to stop taking these medicines. You will also be informed which medicines you can take on the day of your surgery, as well as what time you will need to stop eating and drinking the night before.

Arthroscopy is typically performed as an outpatient procedure. You will go home shortly after your surgery is complete.

Before your surgery, you will meet with an anesthesiologist to discuss your options. Typically, shoulder arthroscopy is performed with a regional nerve block. Your doctor or the anesthesiologist will give you injections of a numbing medication in the base of your neck or in your shoulder. You may also get sedation to keep you comfortable and prevent you from moving during your procedure. You will not feel anything during your surgery, as well as for a few hours afterward. Some procedures are performed using general anesthesia, in which you are unconscious and unable to feel pain.

Once you are in the operating room, you will be placed in one of two positions:

- In the beach chair position, you sit semi-reclined on a chair that looks like a TV lounger, with your head secured in a headrest. This position is used in two-thirds of all shoulder surgeries, including most rotator cuff repairs. It gives your surgeon good access and a clear view of your shoulder. There have been concerns raised in studies about a slightly increased risk of stroke in people who are given general anesthesia and placed in this position, because it may reduce the flow of blood to the brain. Carefully monitoring blood pressure during the procedure and ensuring that it does not drop too low can help prevent this rare complication.
- In the lateral decubitus position, you lie on your side on an operating table. This position gives your surgeon better access to your glenohumeral joint, labrum, and subacromial space. It also puts the sur-

geon's arms in a more comfortable position, which can help prevent fatigue.

In either position, your forearm will likely be placed in a holding device to keep it still. The surgical team will clean the skin of your shoulder with an antiseptic solution. Then the surgeon will inject a saline solution into your shoulder. The fluid expands your shoulder, making it easier for the surgeon to see the internal structures.

The arthroscope will be inserted into your shoulder through a small incision. Images from the scope's camera will appear on a monitor in the operating room, enabling your surgeon to view the procedure as he or she works. The surgeon will make other small incisions and insert the necessary instruments through them.

Types of arthroscopic procedures

Each arthroscopic procedure is performed in a different way. Many of these procedures may be done with open surgery if the damage is too extensive for the surgeon to fix through small incisions.

Rotator cuff repair. To repair a torn rotator cuff, the surgeon first removes any loose or damaged tendon fragments or other debris from around the torn tissue. This is called debridement. Bone spurs may also be removed from the underside of the acromion. Then, the surgeon attaches the torn tendon to its previous position at the top of the humerus, by stitching (suturing) the tendon to metal or plastic anchors placed in the bone.

Labrum repair/removal. First, the surgeon removes the damaged parts of the labrum and any other damaged pieces of cartilage. For small tears, removing damaged tissue may be enough to relieve the problem. For larger tears, the surgeon will repair the labrum, using stitches (sutures) to reattach the labrum tissue to anchors placed in the glenoid bone. Sometimes open surgery is needed for the reattachment part of the procedure. The decision to perform an open repair may be made before the surgery, based on the surgeon's plan and preferences, or during the procedure if the extent of the injury is larger than anticipated.

Bankart repair. A Bankart tear occurs during shoulder dislocation, when the labrum is torn away from the glenoid, causing chronic shoulder instability. This procedure helps to stabilize the shoulder joint after multiple dislocations by putting the ball firmly back into its socket. During this procedure, the surgeon repairs torn ligaments and cartilage. Then the surgeon places small anchors into the bone of the shoulder socket and uses stitches to reattach the labrum. A torn capsule is also repaired.

Debridement. For some people with chronic shoulder pain due to arthritis, simply removing damaged tissue may be enough to relieve the pain. The surgeon removes any bone spurs, damaged cartilage, scar tissue, loose tissue, and other debris that may be pressing on and causing pain in healthy tissues.

SLAP repair. SLAP stands for "superior labrum anterior and posterior." A SLAP tear is a rip in the top part of the labrum, where the biceps tendon attaches to the labrum. During this procedure, the surgeon may reattach the torn portion of the labrum to the bone of the shoulder socket with stitches and anchors or just remove the damaged tissue using debridement. If the biceps tendon is injured, the surgeon may also perform a biceps tenodesis (see below).

Acromioclavicular (AC) joint separation repair. This procedure fixes a severe separation of the AC joint, in which the ligaments that connect the collarbone and scapula are torn, causing the collarbone to move out of position. To repair this, the surgeon brings together the torn ligaments and may use surgical screws, stitches, pins, or other devices to realign and anchor the collarbone in place. Then the damaged ligaments are repaired with stitches.

Shoulder decompression. This procedure treats shoulder impingement syndrome, when the tendons, bursa, or both are trapped by the shoulder bone, restricting movement. The goal of this surgery is to open up a space in the shoulder joint to give the joint room to move. This involves removing the swollen bursa and possibly the coracoacromial ligament. The surgeon will also shave the underside of the acromion bone to leave more space for the rotator cuff tendons.

Biceps tenodesis. Surgeons perform this procedure to treat biceps problems that are due to a SLAP tear or that are caused by inflammation and irritation of the biceps tendon (biceps tendinitis). The two biceps tendons attach the biceps muscle to bones in the shoulder. During this procedure, the surgeon cuts one of the tendons where it attaches to the labrum on the shoulder socket, and reattaches it to the humerus bone, using screws to hold it in place. This relieves pressure on the tendon and helps to ease shoulder pain.

Arthroscopic capsular release. This procedure relieves pain and restores mobility in people with frozen shoulder. The surgeon inserts a probe into the shoulder. The probe releases radiofrequency waves, which make the molecules inside the shoulder tissue move rapidly back and forth (oscillate) and heat up, essentially vaporizing the troublesome scar tissue. This frees up the shoulder, allowing it to move again.

AC joint resection. The surgeon removes a small piece of bone from the end of the collarbone to create space between the collarbone and the end of the acromion. This prevents the collarbone and the acromion bone from rubbing against each other in people with arthritis.

Distal clavicle resection (Mumford procedure). This procedure, which is essentially the same as AC joint resection, is done to relieve pain due to arthritis or impingement syndrome, when the rotator cuff tendons rub painfully against the bottom of the acromion bone. This can eventually weaken or tear the rotator cuff. The surgeon first removes the inflamed bursa sac. Then, the surgeon shaves off or removes a small piece of the outer part of the collarbone to relieve pressure and improve mobility. When there are larger rotator cuff tears, this procedure can be done through an open procedure using a single incision.

Biologic shoulder resurfacing. This minimally invasive procedure is a new alternative for younger (under age 50), active people who have arthritis or other degeneration in the shoulder joint that has not improved with conservative treatments such as physical therapy or steroid injections. Joint replacement is not recommended for such people, because intense activity in the future could loosen the new joint or cause it to fail. If the joint fails, you will have to undergo revision surgery. In biologic resurfacing, the surgeon replaces the worn and damaged cartilage in the shoulder joint with healthy cartilage and bone tissue taken from the shoulder, knee, or ankle of a deceased donor. The advantage is that this procedure uses real human tissue, rather than synthetic metal or plastic as in a traditional shoulder replacement. Because only a small amount of bone is removed, it will be possible for you to have a total shoulder replacement in the future if you need one. (Many people who have this procedure will eventually need a shoulder replacement.) However, because this procedure is still relatively new, long-term data on its effectiveness are not yet available. Also, biologic resurfacing may not be available at every orthopedic center.

After your surgery

After the arthroscopic procedure is completed, your surgeon may close the incisions with stitches or surgical tape and place a bandage on top. The entire procedure generally takes less than an hour. However, everyone's situation is different. Your surgery may be slightly shorter or longer than the average depending on the extent of repairs you need.

If you had general anesthesia, you will need to stay in the recovery room for one to two hours while you awaken from the anesthesia. No matter what kind of anesthesia you have, someone will have to drive you home and stay with you for the first night.

You will be in some discomfort after your procedure. Expect the pain to last for at least a week. Your doctor will send you home from the hospital with a prescription for pain relievers, which can include opioids, NSAIDs, or acetaminophen (Tylenol). Opioids relieve pain effectively, but they can be addictive. If your doctor prescribes these drugs, take them exactly as the label recommends.

During your recovery, be careful to keep your incision clean. You can take a shower once the wounds are no longer draining, but do not scrub your incisions.

Arthroscopy generally leads to a faster recovery than open surgery. However, the length of your recovery depends on the extent of your repair. It can take anywhere from a few days to a few weeks to get back to your previous activities, and up to six months to fully heal. While your shoulder is healing, you may need to wear a sling or immobilizer to keep it still and prevent reinjury.

Open surgery

Arthroscopy has some advantages over open surgery, including a faster recovery and smaller scars. For some types of procedures—including rotator cuff tears—surgeons are moving away from open surgery and increasingly performing them arthroscopically. However, there are situations in which a traditional open incision is necessary, including for larger and more complex shoulder injuries. Today, orthopedic surgeons can perform open procedures through smaller incisions, measuring just an inch or two long. New technologies are improving the safety and outcomes of these procedures even further (see "How technology is reshaping shoulder repair," below).

How technology is reshaping shoulder repair

Technology is transforming every aspect of our lives—from the way we communicate to the tools that we use to stay healthy. Not surprisingly, a number of innovations have made their way into the operating room. The following are just two of the new technologies that are making shoulder surgery easier and safer than ever before.

Virtual reality. Watching surgical procedures or practicing on a dummy or cadaver can't fully prepare medical students for the reality of operating on a live human being. The recent development of virtual reality gives students access to an immersive environment that accurately simulates the operating room setting and specific problems that can occur. Virtual reality provides both visual and tactile feedback to the surgeon, who can practice surgery in much the same way as a pilot uses a simulator to gain the experience of flying a plane. Errors can be made virtually, rather than on a patient, thus improving skills for the real surgical situation. Many companies are developing such technology, which will no doubt play a large role in surgeon training in the future.

Augmented reality. Augmented reality is the practice of superimposing virtual elements onto the real world. We use this technology when we look at a heads-up display on a car windshield. The military has used augmented reality for years as part of its technology for targeting and flying planes. In the medical field, the surgeon wears a special head-mounted digital display similar to Google Glass. Through the display, the doctor can see a three-dimensional projected model of the surgical field on which to map out the surgery step by step. Augmented reality also has an application inside the operating room: virtual guides prevent errors and guide the surgeon.

Types of open surgical procedures

The following procedures are performed through open surgery. These procedures are typically done while you are under general anesthesia, although they may be performed using regional anesthesia or with a combination of the two anesthetic types.

Open rotator cuff repair. Doctors recommend performing a rotator cuff repair as an open procedure if the tear is particularly large or if you have tears in tendons or other soft tissue that also need to be fixed. During this surgery, the surgeon makes one large incision over the shoulder and detaches the deltoid muscle to gain access to the rotator cuff. The surgeon will also remove any bone spurs from the underside of the acromion, a procedure known as an acromioplasty.

Latarjet procedure. This procedure treats shoulder instability that has not been relieved by Bankart repair or another procedure to fix damaged structures. It can be performed arthroscopically, but it is most often done as an open procedure. During the surgery, the surgeon cuts a piece of bone from the coracoid process and drills holes in it. Then, the surgeon shaves the glenoid and attaches the coracoid bone directly to the socket with screws. This creates a kind of sling that stabilizes the shoulder joint and prevents the humerus from dislocating again.

ORIF fracture repair surgery. Open reduction and internal fixation (ORIF) is a procedure that is used to fix a broken humerus. Typically, fractures are treated with more conservative measures, such as a sling and pain medicine. Doctors recommend surgery only if the bone is broken into several pieces, the fragments do not line up correctly, the bone has broken through the skin, or the fracture would not have healed well on its own. ORIF is typically performed as an emergency procedure soon after the injury. The "open" in ORIF refers to the incision the surgeon uses to get to the broken bone. Once the surgeon has placed the bones back into the correct position (the "reduction" step), "fixation" involves the use of screws, stitches, rods, wires, or metal plates to hold the bone in place while it heals.

Total shoulder replacement. When your arthritis pain and stiffness is so severe that conservative treatments like physical therapy and pain relievers have not led to any real improvements, a total shoulder replacement may be the best option for restoring your movement and easing your discomfort (see Figure 9, at left). During this procedure, the surgeon first removes the damaged humeral head and inserts either a stem into the hollow bone of the humerus or a short implant into the broad section of the top of the humerus. This creates the space for the surgeon to see the glenoid socket. The socket is then prepared and resurfaced with a polyethylene (hard plastic) implant, after which the surgeon places a metal ball on the stem or the short implant that was previously inserted in the humerus. The goal is to replicate your original anatomy as closely as possible. Cement may be used to fix the socket, but it is rarely used on the stem in the humerus.

Reverse total shoulder replacement. A traditional shoulder replacement may not be a good option for people with large rotator cuff tears who have developed rotator cuff tear arthropathy (see "Rotator cuff tear," page 20). To move your shoulder joint after a traditional procedure, you will need healthy rotator cuff muscles. If these muscles have been damaged, you may still be left with limited range of motion

Figure 9: Total shoulder replacement

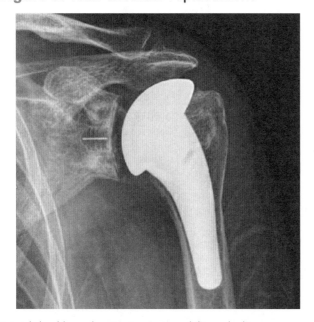

A total shoulder replacement restores mobility and relieves pain caused by severe arthritis of the shoulder joint. During this procedure, the surgeon replaces the damaged joint with a prosthetic metal humerus (ball), which fits into a plastic glenoid (socket).
Image: Dr. Jon J.P. Warner, Harvard Medical School.

after a conventional shoulder joint replacement.

A reverse total shoulder replacement solves this problem by orienting the new joint in the opposite direction from usual. The plastic cup is attached to the upper end of the arm bone rather than the shoulder socket, while the metal ball is screwed into the shoulder socket instead of the arm bone (see Figure 10, at right). The effect is that, instead of the ball moving within the fixed socket, the socket moves around the fixed ball. This places the shoulder prosthesis in a position that allows the deltoid muscle rather than the rotator cuff to stabilize, power, and move the joint.

This procedure may also be appropriate for people who have had a previous total shoulder replacement but who continue to experience pain and limited movement. In this case, the surgery is considered a "revision" to the previous surgery, and the earlier prosthesis must be removed before the new one is implanted. Revision surgery is always more complicated to perform than the original surgery, because of scarring that forms in the soft tissues of the shoulder. If you need revision surgery, ensure that it's done by an experienced surgeon who regularly performs these types of procedures.

Stemless shoulder replacement. Typical shoulder prostheses have a long stem that fits all the way down into the humerus, or arm bone. However, this design comes with a few potential problems. For one thing, the arm bone could potentially break around the prosthesis. And if you were to need revision surgery, it would be very difficult to remove and replace the stem without cutting through the middle of the humerus. The long stem also transfers weight from the shoulder to the arm, which disrupts normal shoulder mechanics. For people with enough remaining bone, a stemless shoulder is a new alternative to the long-stemmed prosthetic. It preserves more of your original bone, and the implant acts more like your natural shoulder would. The surgical results are similar to those of traditional long-stemmed implants, but the surgery is faster and it results in less blood loss and pain. Several companies have developed stemless implants, which have been gaining popularity.

Shoulder resurfacing. Shoulder resurfacing is not performed as often as knee and hip resurfacing, but it is an option for people with arthritis who have

Figure 10: Reverse shoulder replacement

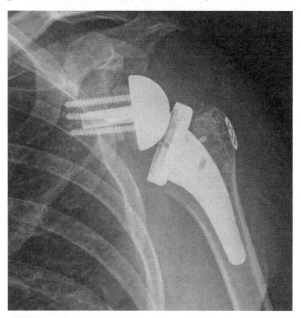

A reverse shoulder replacement places the ball and socket in the opposite positions from where they would naturally be located. The metal ball is attached to the shoulder socket, while the socket is attached to the humerus (upper arm bone).
Image: Dr. Jon J.P. Warner, Harvard Medical School.

enough healthy bone remaining in their joint. Unlike a total shoulder replacement, resurfacing replaces only the surface of the humeral head, the glenoid socket, or both. The damaged surfaces are smoothed over and then covered with a metal prosthetic cap, which is screwed into the bone. Because the surgeon removes less bone from the joint, shoulder resurfacing typically results in less blood loss, fewer complications, and a shorter recovery time than a total replacement. However, it may not be as effective. Traditional shoulder replacement surgery remains the gold standard for providing long-term pain relief.

After open shoulder surgery

You may need to stay in the hospital for two to three days after your surgery. Each person is unique, and the length of your stay will depend on the type of procedure you had and the speed of your recovery. You will receive pain medicine while in the hospital and to take home with you.

Cryotherapy (cold therapy) is another important pain-relieving method, and it can help reduce your reliance on pain medications while you heal. Cryotherapy typically involves the use of either an ice pack or a cold therapy unit. Cryocuff is one type of cold therapy unit that circulates cold throughout your joint via a wrap that you wear around your shoulder. It is more efficient at delivering cold than a traditional ice pack would be, but it is also more expensive. Game Ready is another type of cold therapy unit. Along with the cold, it alternately delivers compression to the surgical site to reduce swelling after surgery.

You will wear a sling on your arm for four to six weeks after your surgery to protect the area while it heals. During this time, practice the exercises your doctor or physical therapist taught you (you will need to first remove the sling). The first exercises you will likely do are to make a fist, move your fingers, and bend and straighten your elbow. These actions help to prevent stiffness in the arm, elbow, and hand and keep your blood flowing normally.

It may take up to six weeks for you to fully resume your normal activities—including driving. How soon you can return to work depends on the type of job you have. You will be able to return to a desk job sooner than you would to a position that requires more physical exertion. Your doctor will let you know when it is safe and appropriate for you to go back to your regular activities, including exercise. Don't expect to be back on the field throwing fastballs two weeks after your surgery. Starting too soon could lead to injury, and it could undermine everything you—and your surgeon—have worked to accomplish. It could take a few months before you can return to sports and exercise. You should eventually make a full return to sports that don't involve the risk of contact or collision. Activities like tennis, golf, and swimming are typically fine. You may want to avoid sports in which you could fall and damage your new joint, such as skiing.

During your recovery, you will have regularly scheduled visits with your orthopedic surgeon, who will make sure that the surgical site is healing properly. Expect to see your doctor at regular intervals—one week, two weeks, six weeks, three months, six months, and one year after your procedure. The number and frequency of your follow-up visits will be determined by the type of surgery you had and how quickly you

are healing. It's important that you stick to the recovery plan your doctor prescribes and complete your physical therapy as directed (see "Post-surgery rehabilitation," below). Failing to do your part after surgery could mean you don't get the best possible results.

Possible complications

Shoulder surgery is typically very successful. Many people who undergo one of these procedures are able to return to their previous activities with a significant reduction in pain.

Yet any surgery comes with risks. Most people will have at least some pain and stiffness following their procedure. Serious complications are rare, and the introduction of new surgical techniques has reduced the likelihood of having a significant problem after surgery. Following are the most common risks from shoulder surgery:

- infection (signs include a fever over 101° F, redness, drainage from the wound, and warmth)
- excessive bleeding
- increased pain or swelling
- blood clots
- shoulder weakness
- injury to a nearby blood vessel or nerve
- numbness or tingling in the arm or hand
- shoulder instability or dislocation
- in the case of total shoulder replacement, loosening of the prosthesis (approximately 3% of shoulders loosen in 10 years).

Arthroscopy tends to result in less blood loss and pain, as well as fewer complications, compared with open surgery.

Post-surgery rehabilitation

On the day after your surgery, you will meet with your orthopedic surgeon or a physical therapist. Depending on what type of surgery you had, he or she might get you started with some exercises to help regain movement in your shoulder. In other cases, you may have to wait up to six weeks to begin. You will continue to do the exercises at home—both on your own, and during visits with a physical therapist once or twice a week.

As you progress, more exercises will be added to your rehabilitation program, which should include both flexibility or stretching to restore full range of motion in your shoulder, and strength training to bolster the muscles that stabilize and support your shoulder. The exercises your doctor or physical therapist recommends should work all the muscles in your shoulder—deltoid, trapezius, rhomboids, biceps, etc. And your program should be adjusted for any limitations you might have due to your injury or the surgery you had to repair it. For example, if you had rotator cuff repair, you may have to wait for three months to start doing strengthening exercises.

Moving your repaired shoulder will likely feel awkward or painful at first. Yet you need to stick with the exercises your doctor and physical therapist prescribe. Unless you are instructed to keep your arm in a sling, keeping your arm still for a prolonged period could make it stiff and immobile, defeating the purpose of your surgery. The exercises will get easier as you do them, and you will gradually regain strength and mobility in your shoulder.

You should also meet with an occupational therapist, either before you leave the hospital or soon after you return home. This therapist will teach you shortcuts and tips for doing everyday tasks. For example, wear loose-fitting, button-down shirts, and put the arm that was operated on in the sleeve first to make the other arm do most of the work. A long-handled sponge will make it easier to wash your back in the shower, while a grabbing tool will help you reach a box of cereal from a high shelf. Propping a pillow or foam wedge under your shoulder can make sleep more comfortable.

Ease back into your normal daily routine as instructed by your medical team. You will be able to start using your arm for everyday activities, such as dressing and bathing, typically within the first few days or weeks following your surgery, although some surgeries require more time for tissue healing. Your doctor or physical therapist can help guide you through this recovery period. He or she should also let you know when it is safe for you to start a regular exercise program again, what types of exercises are most appropriate given your injury, and how to gradually ramp up to increase strength and flexibility in the affected shoulder. You will likely be cleared to use a stationary bike or take walks on a treadmill within days following your surgery. You may not be cleared to return to more strenuous activities such as running, swimming, and tennis for four to six months, so be sure to discuss this with your surgeon before resuming these activities.

At the same time, for up to six months after your surgery, you will typically continue physical therapy. However, it's a good idea to keep doing the exercises two or three times a week afterward on your own to maintain strength and flexibility in the shoulder joint. It may take as much as one to two years for the shoulder to fully recover after surgery.

Preventing future shoulder problems

Once your shoulder has fully healed, you still need to be mindful about how you use this joint to avoid another injury. To ward off future problems, follow the advice given earlier in this report on proper posture and form. Set up an ergonomic workstation. And be careful how you lift heavy objects—to protect not just your back, but your shoulders, too. In addition, follow these tips:

Know your limits. Do not try to push your shoulder past its capabilities. Gradually return to sports and other activities, and don't do anything more strenuous than your doctor recommends. If you play a sport that requires you to repeatedly throw or swing, be careful. Repetitive movements can re-damage the structures that have just recently healed. If you are engaged in throwing or lifting activities and you ever feel a twinge or real pain, stop what you are doing. For pain that is severe or continuous, see your doctor right away.

Exercise consistently, but safely. Keep doing the shoulder exercises your physical therapist recommended, paying special attention to any tips you've been given on maintaining correct form. You should also have a regular regimen of aerobic and strengthening exercises. Make sure to warm up for five to 10 minutes before you start exercising. Take the same amount of time to cool down afterward.

Take regular breaks during the day. Get up from your chair about once every 30 minutes. Walk around, do a few shoulder rolls, shake out your arms, and stretch your muscles. ▼

Resources

Organizations

American Academy of Orthopaedic Surgeons/American Association of Orthopaedic Surgeons (AAOS)
9400 W. Higgins Road
Rosemont, IL 60018
847-823-7186
www.aaos.org

AAOS represents two organizations that act in the interests of orthopedic surgeons around the world. The Academy is the educational arm; it provides continuing medical education to orthopedic surgeons. The Association engages in health policy and advocacy efforts on behalf of people working in this medical specialty. The website offers a tool that lets patients find an orthopedist by specialty and location.

American College of Radiology (ACR)
1891 Preston White Drive
Reston, VA 20191
703-648-8900
www.acr.org

The American College of Radiology represents nearly 40,000 radiologists and other specialists in this field. One of its main missions is to advance the science and delivery of radiology care. The ACR's patient-centered website (www.radiologyinfo.org), co-sponsored with the Radiological Society of North America, provides background information on a variety of diagnostic imaging techniques.

American College of Rheumatology
2200 Lake Blvd. NE
Atlanta, GA 30319
404-633-3777
www.rheumatology.org

This national organization of rheumatology professionals advocates on behalf of patients with arthritis and the practitioners who treat them. It also hosts an annual meeting, which highlights the latest research on arthritis and other musculoskeletal diseases.

Arthritis Foundation
1355 Peachtree St. NE, Suite 600
Atlanta, GA 30309
404-872-7100
www.arthritis.org

The Arthritis Foundation pushes for research toward new treatments and ultimately a cure for arthritis. This organization also provides information and resources—including support groups and exercise programs—for people who are living with all forms of this disease.

Boston Shoulder Institute
55 Fruit St., Suite 3G, 3200
Boston, MA 02114
617-724-7300
www.bostonshoulderinstitute.com

Boston Shoulder Institute is the practice of Dr. Jon J.P. Warner, the medical editor of this report. The practice provides state-of-the-art care for shoulder problems, based on the latest clinical research. It offers an extensive website, with descriptions of common shoulder conditions and procedures and personal stories from patients.

National Institute of Arthritis and Musculoskeletal and Skin Diseases (NIAMS)
National Institutes of Health
Bldg. 31, Room 4C02
31 Center Drive, MSC 2350
Bethesda, MD 20892
301-496-8190
www.niams.nih.gov

NIAMS supports research into the causes and treatment of musculoskeletal diseases like arthritis. The organization also provides information to help people with these conditions make better decisions about their own health.

Harvard Health Publications

Other Special Health Reports from Harvard Medical School elaborate on some of the themes in this report. To order, go to www.health.harvard.edu or call 877-649-9457 (toll-free).

The Joint Pain Relief Workout: Healing exercises for your shoulders, hips, knees, and ankles
Lauren E. Elson, M.D., Medical Editor, and Michele Stanten, Fitness Consultant
(Harvard Medical School, 2018)
In addition to the shoulder workout, which is reprinted here in *Healing Shoulder Pain,* there are workouts for other major joints.

Living Well with Osteoarthritis: A guide to keeping your joints healthy
Robert H. Shmerling, M.D., Medical Editor
(Harvard Medical School, 2019)
Osteoarthritis—the most common type of arthritis—is painful and can interfere with your ability to do things you enjoy. But there are many steps you can take to protect your joints, reduce discomfort, and improve mobility. This report covers the gamut, from established medical therapies to the use of assistive devices and complementary treatments such as acupuncture.

Neck Pain: A troubleshooting guide to help you relieve your pain, restore function, and prevent injury
Robert H. Shmerling, M.D., Medical Editor
(Harvard Medical School, 2016)
This report covers the most common causes of neck pain, outlines today's treatment options, and provides many simple steps you can take to ease and manage your aches and pains.

Rheumatoid Arthritis: How to protect your joints, reduce pain, and improve mobility
Robert H. Shmerling, M.D., Medical Editor
(Harvard Medical School, 2018)
This report explains the steps you can take to protect your joints, reduce discomfort, and improve your mobility. Because living with this disease involves more than finding a drug treatment, a Special Section provides advice about how to care for yourself through adaptations in your personal and work life.